LADIES, WE

EVERYTHING WE'RE ~~NOT~~ SAYING ABOUT
BODIES, HEALTH, SEX & RELATIONSHIPS

NEED

YUMI STYNES & TO
CLAUDINE RYAN

TALK

WITH ILLUSTRATIONS BY GRACE LEE

Hardie Grant

BOOKS

★ CONTENTS ★

LADIES,
WE
NEED
TO
TALK

Dearest reader,

In this book we're going to explore adult content and themes. While we have thought carefully about everything included in this book, some of the language and stories may offend some people.

Much love,
YUMI & CLAUDINE

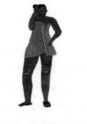

★ INTRODUCTION ★

YUMI

When Claudine Ryan approached me to be involved in a podcast she was pitching at the ABC, we had never met before. The podcast didn't even have a name. I had never worked for the ABC. Claudine had never made a podcast. It seemed far-fetched, but the two of us met in a cafe and stirred our coffees and talked about the things that stirred our passions.

In 20 years of working in media, I've learnt that you never know where those first meetings are going to go. Often nothing comes of it – the meeting is like a seed that was planted but never grew. A lot of seeds get thrown around in any creative process, and it's hard to predict which are going to die, and which will land and grow into something extraordinary.

If you want to talk growth, it would be difficult to explain the difference between the person I was back then, sitting in that cafe, and who I am now. Suffice to say, the changes have been immense, positive, and I owe a lot of it to Claudine and the hard-working team behind *Ladies, We Need To Talk*. Together, we planted a forest. A lot of the growth was in the work, which you can see and touch and hold in this book. And a lot of it was *here* (I'm pointing to my heart).

When the first episode of the podcast dropped back in September 2017, it immediately found a massive audience. It felt like we'd cracked the code and created a podcast that spoke to listeners in that same precious way that women can speak to each other when they feel safe. You know that kind of talk? Where the tone and volume drops, you check behind you to make sure no-one is listening ... and then you share. Women share confidences. We reveal secrets. We do it with love. And we do it with trust.

Trust is like friendship: it can't be rushed. In those early days, Claudine and I didn't know each other but we caught a good vibe, and we started our work together respectfully and with kindness. That has extended to everything we've done with the podcast, including this book. And it includes how we want to treat you: our listener and reader.

Working on the podcast put me in regular contact with a suite of amazing and accomplished ladies and sometimes even made me feel like I could be one of them. From experts to survivors, regular people with a story to tell, those who have endured shocking trauma, and doctors and professors who have changed lives, I've learnt so much from everyone we have interviewed.

Crucially, I've learnt that being awesome is a daily practice – like meditating or parenting or training for a marathon. You have to keep at it, and it's being dogged and determined and savagely committed that makes you unreal.

CLAUDINE

I went to Yumi Stynes with a seed of an idea; we planted and grew it together. The idea was simple: create a podcast by women for women where we'd explore things we feel uncomfortable talking about. Things like peeing ourselves when we exercise, discharge that bleaches our undies, sex that hurts or feels like a job to cross off your to-do list, or the kind of toe-curling sex you fantasise about.

In my work as a health reporter and digital editor for the ABC, I had learnt that there was a big audience for stories about these kinds of 'taboo' topics. I had read enough research and interviewed plenty of experts who helped me understand there was a real knowledge gap when it came to women's health and sexuality, and hiding in this gap were things women needed to know. I wanted women to know that one in two women over 50 who have been pregnant experience prolapse, but what you do when you're younger can reduce the risk. More than 70 per cent of women over 40 have low libido, and this doesn't have to mean your sex life is over forever. Women are more likely to be dissatisfied with their body than not, but just knowing this can be the first step in starting to challenge unrealistic beauty standards in your own way. Those of us in heterosexual relationships are getting ripped off when it comes to orgasms during sex with their partner, but you can make your pleasure a priority.

Soon after making contact with Yumi, I discovered that she was exactly the kind of woman I wanted to work with – smart, funny, fearless, hard-working, as well as big-hearted, practical and thoughtful. Just before our first phone conversation I had been caught in torrential downpour, and as we spoke I was shivering in wet clothes in the ABC Ultimo office. Ten minutes after we hung up, I got a text from Yumi – she'd dropped off a dry change of clothes for me at reception. I fell for her then and knew our audience would too. She was like the cool best friend I had wanted in high school, one who would encourage me to go outside my comfort zone, but who looked out for me and would always have my back.

When we finally met for coffee, Yumi and I talked about many things, including how sex education totally lets down girls (and boys). Outside school, the lack of knowledge and shame in talking about 'private parts' crosses generations. The impact of this lack of knowledge and confidence in talking about our bodies is that far too often we don't know our bodies, and we don't know ourselves.

We spoke about how so many of us shy away from our own bodies. We don't know how they work. We don't know how to get the help we need when something is wrong. We don't know how to advocate for ourselves with our partners and doctors.

We wanted to empower women – our listeners and now our readers – with the right language. We wanted to help them build confidence and to let them know that they aren't alone, that their bodies aren't gross and that for every shameful, embarrassing secret being kept under wraps, there is an antidote called knowledge. And knowledge often leads to power.

There's this idea that women talk with each other about everything, but there are actually still some big no-go zones. Sometimes they're so taboo they've become invisible to us. Sometimes we won't talk about them because we feel uncomfortable, or don't want to offend or hurt someone's feelings. We made a decision for the podcast to head right into those no-go zones. In this book, we've focused on the no-go zones that make us feel the MOST uncomfortable and most urgently need to be talked about.

For some of you these conversations may make you feel awkward, even squeamish. But that's OK – it's what happens when you do something new. Truth is, if you are a grown-up, with a grown-up body, who enjoys doing grown-up things, then you need to know your body. Get to know its names. Find out what it likes and dislikes. Maybe even give it a smile from time to time.

The *Ladies* team has always wanted to put out a book because we wanted to go a little deeper. To take the time and space to lay out facts and stories in a way that you could come back to and double-check and re-read. This stuff is real, and it takes longer than a podcast episode to sink in. Also sometimes you need to see something for it to truly make sense, so it's been a joy to be able to include beautiful diagrams and illustrations.

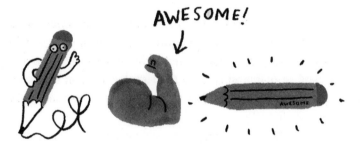

From very soon after we first decided to pitch the podcast, and throughout the journey of *Ladies, We Need To Talk*, the podcast and now the book, we've worked with many other women. Smart, amazing, talented women with skills, knowledge and lived experiences. They shared the same commitment to our audience – the same commitment to empowering women through knowledge and a sense of connection. None of this would have been possible without them.

One of the central tenets of both the podcast and this book is that we only include the voices of women, gender non-conforming and non-binary people. But EVERYONE is welcome. Pass this book on to special people in your life – guys included. We think there are a lot of men who will benefit from reading it. (And if you're a woman who's partnered with a man? Bookmark the bits he needs to read. Trust us, there'll be some things!)

Everyone who worked with us on *Ladies, We Need To Talk* hoped that when women were given the space to respectfully share stories about their experiences, they would feel less alone. That's exactly the feedback we have had. Our listeners have sent so many emails, text messages and voice memos and reached out on social media. They have shared their stories because they want to feel less alone. They have been willing to open up the most private parts of their lives to us because they want other women to know they are not alone. To go full circle and bring those listeners' voices into this book and share them with a whole new audience has been thrilling and emotional.

One of our favourite contributors (and the very first person we interviewed) is Dr Melissa Kang, who was *the* legendary Dolly Doctor for more than 23 years. (She and Yumi have gone on to write bestselling books together.) Dr Kang had a unique insight into the deepest and most secretly held fears of young women through the letters she received. She says, 'Probably the most frequently asked question to Dolly Doctor in 23 years is, "Am I normal?"'

Something that has defined *Ladies, We Need To Talk* is this idea of being 'normal'. It has come up in pretty much every conversation we have had with experts on the show, and it's at the heart of many of our deepest, quietest fears.

The following story about Louise and Madi sums up so much of what *Ladies, We Need To Talk* is all about – the fact that there is no such thing as normal, the difficulty that remains for women to get proper health treatments, and the power of talking!

For more than 40 years, Louise knew something didn't feel quite right in her body. As a teenager her periods were painful and tampons didn't work. She'd put one in, but blood would still find its way onto her underpants.

'At a very young age it changed the course of my life – I wanted to swim competitively, but [because tampons didn't work] I couldn't train fully. Doctors and gynos kept telling me I wasn't changing tampons often enough. But I was. And I just remember actually yelling at one of the specialists, saying in innocence, "It's like I've got two of them!"'

Louise's mum took her to a gynaecologist, who told her 'everything was normal, everything was fine'. Soon after, she changed doctors and her new GP did some tests and found that she had endometriosis. But still tampons didn't work for her.

'When I started having pain through intercourse and I eventually went to another gynaecologist, he said, "I think it's all in your head. You need to go and see a psychiatrist." So I dutifully went off to the psychiatrist. And that was sort of it.

'It was just frustrating because I was pretty sure it wasn't in my head, but then I was starting to doubt myself as well.'

After that she stayed away from gynaecologists and lived with the pain.

So we're talking about 40 years of pain and no diagnosis – until a few years ago, in her mid-50s, when a friend encouraged Louise to go and see *her* gyno. 'She said, "She specialises in women." And I said, "Well, isn't that what gynaecologists do?" And she said, "Yes, but she *really* specialises in things."'

Louise finally found out what was happening: she had two reproductive systems. 'I was born with two of everything. I've got two vaginal cavities – side by side, the left and right, sort of thing.' Two vaginas, two uteruses, two cervixes, but only one set of ovaries. This explains why she would still leak even with a tampon in – it was only capturing blood from *one* vagina/uterus, but not the other.

This unique set-up is called *uterus didelphys*, and it's difficult to detect if you don't know what you're looking for. In Louise's case, she tended to 'favour' one vagina over the other. 'The thing is that you don't feel it, but you feel pain. And that's why sometimes when I was having Pap smears I'd absolutely hit the roof because they'd gone up the one that was hardly ever used.'

Louise has only recently started telling her friends about having uterus didelphys. 'That's what made me decide to contact you. Not one of my friends had heard of this or even knew it could exist. I thought, "Well, if they've got daughters – what if they've gone through something like this and they've just never found out or talked about it?"'

Louise's experience was featured on our 'Secret Lives of Vaginas' episode, and when a listener called Madi heard it, everything fell into place.

Because of that episode, I went to a doctor because I finally realised there was a name for what I have and that I wasn't imagining it. I've been diagnosed with bicornuate bicollis uterus with two vaginas – a malformation a lot like Louise's which means I have two vaginas, two cervixes and two uterus cavities. I never knew what was different about me before that episode, and I might never have known if I hadn't heard the episode with Louise. – **MADI**

It's a perfect example of why we wanted to publish this book. Sharing our stories can be *so* powerful. Too often women have had their experiences dismissed. They have been told it's in their head or just part of being a woman. But when you hear that others have had a similar experience to yours, then it can help you to keep pushing for the answers you need.

We wanted to give the right of reply to our listeners: the *Ladies* community. Because, although when it comes to our bodies, our relationships and the state of our hearts, no two experiences are the same, the more voices we include, the more likely you are to find the words you need to describe your own unique experience.

We hope the words, information and experiences that you find in this book give you confidence. We hope they give you power. The power to talk to your partner about how and where you want to be touched (it's not trivial). The power to talk to your doctor confidently about what is happening with your body and not be dismissed or gaslit when they can't figure out the answer. The power that comes from knowing *this is my body* and *I know it best*.

We hope that once you have realised your power, you may inspire others to find theirs.

If you're ever feeling ashamed for reasons that are impossible to describe, if you're ever feeling confused or gaslit, if you're ever feeling alone or like you might not be 'normal' ... well, ladies, we need to talk.

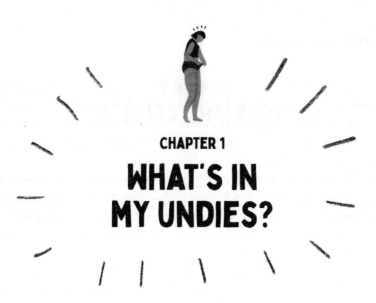

CHAPTER 1
WHAT'S IN MY UNDIES?

A midwife once offered Yumi a mirror in case she wanted to look at her vulva. Yumi's polite response was, 'No thanks.' But in her mind she was hollering (in an over-the-top Scottish brogue): *WHAT, WOMAN? Are you MAD? Why would I want to look at that nightmare right after giving birth? I already know what roadkill looks like!*

Living with a continuous, low-key hum of disgust for female genitals is pretty common among a lot of women. It can manifest in a million ways, like the need to always shower before sex, or to manipulate our laundry so our partner is never confronted with the smear of discharge on our undies. You hear it in comments like, 'I'd love to be a lesbian but I could never go down on a woman. Ugggggh!' or people describing the smell of vaginas as 'fishy' – and not in a good-Japanese-sushi kind of way. And some of the worst insults in the English language refer directly to ... well, you know.

The impact of these taboos is that there's a huge knowledge gap about our bodies and how they work.

This ignorance or confusion isn't something to feel ashamed or embarrassed about – it's as common and perplexing as that sprinkling of sand at the bottom of your handbag. Research by YouGov UK in 2019 found that **52 per cent of the 2000 people surveyed couldn't locate the vagina on a diagram nor explain its function.** Forty-seven per cent couldn't locate the labia, and an astounding 58 per cent didn't know where to find the urethra. As well as not knowing the location of female body parts on a diagram, we frequently misname them. For starters, the vulva and vagina are NOT the same thing!

Ladies, we need to talk about WHAT'S IN OUR UNDIES.

A VERY IMPORTANT REFRESH

The word *vagina* is often used to describe everything inside our undies, but that's wrong. The vagina is the tubular muscle that connects your uterus to the outside world. The parts of your genitals that you can see on the outside of your body make up your *vulva*. It wasn't until Claudine was 28 and had given birth to her first kid that she used the word vulva in a sentence and knew that she was using it correctly.

The fact that so many of us are misnaming such crucial body parts is a fascinating disaster. It's important. And yet we're getting it wrong en masse.

So ... let's get a refresh!

WHAT YOU SEE
(FROM THE OUSIDE)

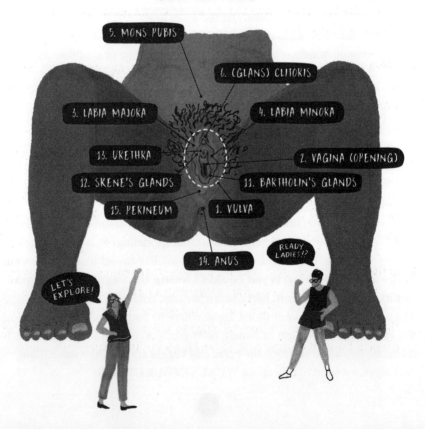

1. **VULVA** This is all the parts of the female genitalia found on the outside of the body. It includes the clitoris, inner and outer labia, and openings of the urethra and vagina. The first known use of the word is from the 14th century and likely came from the word 'volvo', which means to turn or wrap around.

2. **VAGINA** The stretchy muscular tube that connects the uterus to outside the body. At one end is the cervix and at the other is the vaginal opening on the vulva. The vagina is where the penis, fingers and sex toys go during sex; where a baby passes through during childbirth; and where menstrual blood flows through during a period. While the vagina has nerve endings and is sensitive, particularly towards the opening, for most people with one, it isn't really 'action central' when it comes to pleasure. The earliest known reference to the vagina was in 1612 and it comes from the Latin word for 'scabbard or sheath'.

3. **LABIA MAJORA** Also known as the outer labia, the labia majora are the outer fatty flaps of the vulva that are covered with pubic hair. Labia majora is Latin for 'larger lips'.

4. **LABIA MINORA** Latin for 'smaller lips', the labia minora, also known as the inner labia, are the hairless inner lips of the vulva. The labia minora sit inside the labia majora, but their length varies, so the outer reaches of the labia minora can protrude and be seen beyond the labia majora.

5. **MONS PUBIS** This pad of fatty tissue sits above the vulva, on the outside of the pubic symphysis (which is where the pubic bones join together in the front). Mons is Latin for 'mountain', and this area used to be known as the *mons veneris*, which was the Latin for 'mountain of Venus' (the Roman goddess of love).

6. **CLITORIS** If you have a clitoris then this is probably your pleasure epicentre. It sits at the top of your vulva, above your urethra. Much of the clitoris is internal – the only visible part on the outside, the glans clitoris, is just the tip of the clit-berg. There's so much to say about the clitoris that we've devoted the next chapter to it, so buckle up 'cos there's plenty to come!

THE FEMALE REPRODUCTIVE SYSTEM
(FROM THE FRONT)

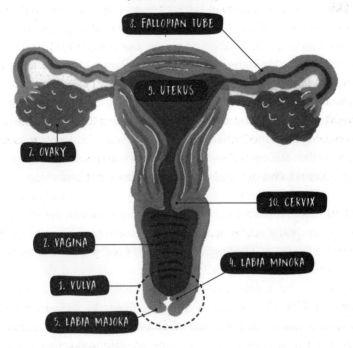

8. FALLOPIAN TUBE

9. UTERUS

7. OVARY

10. CERVIX

2. VAGINA

4. LABIA MINORA

1. VULVA

5. LABIA MAJORA

7. **OVARIES** These two small almond-shaped glands produce ova (eggs) and reproductive hormones (oestrogen and progesterone). Ovaries are the primary sex organs or gonads in females (the male equivalent is the testes or balls). Each month, an ovum (egg) is released by one of the ovaries in a process known as ovulation. The ovum (egg) then travels to the uterus via the fallopian tubes, where it may be fertilised by sperm. The ovaries are a key driver of the menstrual cycle and form an interconnected feedback system with the pituitary gland and the hypothalamus. The name is derived from the Latin *ovum*, meaning ... egg. (You'll read more about ovaries in the chapter on hormones.)

8. **FALLOPIAN TUBES** These tubes run from each side of your uterus to the ovaries. They carry ova (eggs) on the first part of their journey from the ovaries to the uterus, and are the site where fertilisation most often occurs (NOT in your uterus, which is a common misconception). This is one of many parts of the female anatomy named for the man who first described them in texts. Gabriele Falloppio was an Italian Catholic priest, physician and anatomist renowned for his work on reproductive organs (and the ear) in the early 1500s.

9. **UTERUS** This muscular organ is the size and shape of a pear and sits in the lower abdomen. When a sperm fertilises an ovum (egg), this is where the embryo (fertilised egg) will implant. The uterus has three layers that make up the uterine wall: the endometrium, myometrium and perimetrium. During each menstrual cycle, the endometrium thickens in preparation for an embryo to implant itself and then grow and develop into a fetus. If that doesn't happen, the endometrium is shed during the period. The uterus is also sometimes called the womb. The Greek word for womb, *hystera*, is the origin of the word hysteria – originally a 'nervous disease' that was thought to be unique to women and caused by diseases of the uterus.

10. **CERVIX** This cylinder-shaped neck of tissue connects the uterus to the vagina. It produces cervical mucus that changes in consistency during the menstrual cycle and is a key component of our vaginal discharge (much more on discharge from page 20). During menstruation, the cervix opens a small amount to permit the passage of menstrual flow. You can feel the southern end of the cervix by putting your fingers in your vagina and going as far back as you can. Some say it feels a little like the tip of your nose. The cervix is usually closed, long and firm, but during pregnancy it starts to soften. In the lead-up to birth it gets shorter and dilates widely to allow the baby to pass from the uterus through to the vagina.

11. **BARTHOLIN'S GLANDS** These two pea-sized glands sit to the left and right of your vaginal opening and release the fluid that lubricates your vagina when you're feeling horny. These glands were named after the bloke who first described them, which in this case was the Danish anatomist Caspar Bartholin the Younger in the 17th century.

12. **SKENE'S GLANDS** These are found above your vaginal opening on the lower end of the urethra and are believed to be the source of the fluid released if there's vaginal ejaculation during an orgasm. This used to be called squirting, but experts now say squirting is urine expelled from the urethra during orgasm, whereas ejaculation involves smaller amounts of urine as well as a milky white liquid secreted from the Skene's glands. This is another vulvar territory named after a dude: Alexander Skene.

13. **URETHRA** This is your wee hole. It is a thin, short, muscular tube that goes from your bladder to your vulva. The entrance sits below the clitoris and above the vagina. A little like a quiet but highly valued member of your friendship group, the urethra is not as tingly and exciting as the clitoris, nor as open to exploration as the vagina, but you wouldn't want to be without it.

14. **ANUS** This is the sphincter where your poo comes out. What makes a sphincter more interesting than just a regular opening or hole is that it's actually a ring-shaped muscle that relaxes to open a passage or tightens to close it. It's not technically part of your vulva, but it's helpful to know exactly where it sits. Your anus has lots of sensitive nerve endings so some of us get a lot of pleasure from anal stimulation.

15. **PERINEUM** This is the area between the vagina and the anus. Many of us never hear the word 'perineum' until after childbirth when it is paired with the word (deep breath in) 'tear'. It can be extremely sensitive to touch and may be an erogenous zone.

HOW IT ALL FITS
(FROM THE SIDE)

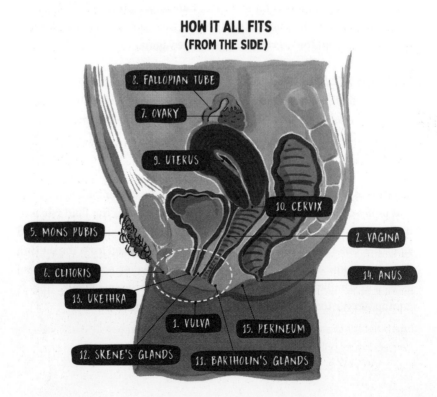

Here's a question we're going to be talking about, a lot. Am I NORMAL? And in this particular case: is what's inside MY underpants normal?

It's what we all worry about, even though we don't even know what normal *is*. We're frightened that we might be monstrous in how we look or smell, how we taste, just by the sheer filth of being in possession of a pussy.

Dr Elizabeth Farrell is one of the many incredible female health professionals we've spoken to while making *Ladies, We Need To Talk*. A gynaecologist and medical director at Jean Hailes for Women's Health in Victoria, Dr Farrell has been awarded an Order of Australia for her decades of work in women's health.

Dr Farrell wants us to understand that despite our similarities, each of us is as unique and distinct as a fingerprint.

'Our periods will not be the same as any other woman's. Our experience of having sex and intercourse will not be the same as anybody else's. Our vulva will look different from everybody else's, and there's a range of normal. You don't have to have a particular shape to be normal.'

Dr Farrell wants you to be PROUD of your vulva and vagina. 'It's about talking about our bodies and being proud of our anatomy, being proud of the fact that as women we have different anatomical parts [from men] as part of our reproductive system. We should love them. We shouldn't abuse them.

'Being happy with your body means that you're able to touch your body and that it's not something to be shameful of. It's something to be proud of.'

Dr Melissa Kang says 'the main message is that all vaginas, vulvas, labia, hymens are different. So there is no one-size-fits-all – literally.'

As I was growing up, no-one told me that vaginal discharge was a thing. I kinda always thought something was wrong with me. When I got into my teenage years and the internet was a thing, I thought I had thrush! But I was too ashamed to talk to anyone about it.

I had a very funny interaction with my husband recently concerning vaginal discharge. We were having a conversation about masturbation, and during it he accused me of being a chronic masturbator! I mean, I do flick the bean quite a lot, but I asked him where he got this idea into his head. He immediately pointed straight to the dirty washing basket and told me to look at all the stuff in the crotch of my underwear. I burst out laughing! He thought my normal daily vaginal discharge was 'lady jizz'. We sat down and I had to educate him on the goings on of vaginas after that! – **SHANNON**

Of all the things that happen inside our underwear, one that freaks many of us out is DISCHARGE. As a teenager, Yumi was in such an information desert that she contemplated writing to Dolly Doctor about it. It felt like the ultimate taboo. No-one talked about it – unless it was in relation to thrush. We never read about it in the hallowed pages of *Cosmopolitan* or *Cleo*, even though they were meant to be for the sexually adventurous. In sex ed we were taught about wet dreams – something that happens to boys – in a way that normalised them and made us feel tolerant and supportive of those who experienced them ... but there was not a peep about discharge. Not. A. Peep.

EVERYONE with a vagina has vaginal discharge. It's as everyday and rudimentary – and normal – as having hair in your nostrils.

Discharge is also marvellous. It keeps your vagina healthy. It helps lubricate your vagina so that sexual activity doesn't hurt and in fact feels fantastic (we're going to talk about this a LOT in the chapter on painful sex). It works as a protective shield that helps to keep vaginal infections at bay.

> This is something that is never spoken about, but has always been a reality for me. I have had vaginal discharge every single day probably since I underwent puberty (I'm now 30). It's not a big amount, but enough that I wear panty liners every day. (And when I have a big day or event, or I do intense exercise, I slip in a tampon just so I don't have to worry about it.) – **SARAH**

Dr Deborah Bateson is the medical director of Family Planning New South Wales and knows all there is to know about discharge. Of all the experts we've interviewed in more than five years of access to brilliant keepers of fascinating information, Dr Bateson was the one we probably had the *most* questions for.

Firstly, Dr Bateson wants to reassure you that 'vaginal discharge is normal, and it's normal to have a bit of odour associated with it'.

Discharge contains a combination of mucus, dead skin cells and vaginal bacteria. It has a characteristic, but inoffensive, smell (which may be stronger in some women due to sweat glands in the pubic area), and is usually clear, creamy or slightly yellow in colour. Your discharge changes in colour, consistency and volume throughout your menstrual cycle, as your hormones change.

'During the cycle ... discharge starts off as dry and sticky,' explains Dr Bateson. 'As we approach ovulation and there is an increase in oestrogen, the discharge changes consistency and becomes a bit milky, stretchy and slippery. After ovulation and we pass the fertile phase, you get a decrease in oestrogen and an increase in progesterone, and the mucus changes again to become thick and sticky.'

There are also certain times during your reproductive life when there will be noticeable changes to your discharge. For instance during pregnancy, when oestrogen levels are higher, there is an increase in the volume of discharge. You'll notice you have less discharge when you have lower oestrogen levels, such as during the postnatal period, perimenopause or after menopause.

Vaginal dryness is a very common feature of menopause and its impact can be devastating. 'We know after menopause that the amount of lubrication decreases and that can be incredibly painful for some women,' says Dr Bateson. For some women the level of discomfort is so significant that they experience pain while they are just walking around. Many of the experts we spoke to wished that people experiencing vaginal dryness knew of the benefits of vaginal oestrogen treatments and asked us to encourage readers to discuss this with their GPs.

Dr Bateson says if she were to line up 10 women, no two would have the same discharge. 'Some of them may be using contraceptives. Some will have recently just had sex and that will have an effect. Some will be menstruating, some won't be. Some may have more sweat glands on the hair-bearing areas than others.'

This is why experts say there is no normal, but Dr Bateson says we all need to know 'our own normal' so we can spot when something has gone awry. Which it does! If we have thrush, certain STIs, bacterial vaginosis, or even a reaction to soaps and cleaning products, our body can react with a hefty discharge that sometimes comes with a foul-smelling odour and/or almighty itching. This is *not* normal – and a good sign to get help.

We also need to know what's normal so that we don't fall prey to messages and misinformation peddled by the feminine hygiene and wellness industries.

Like so many of the other incredibly well-credentialed and thoroughly experienced experts we've spoken to, Dr Bateson is not happy that we're bombarded with advertising and messages telling us to 'stay fresh' inside our undies. Not only are feminine hygiene products – such as intimate washes, wipes and deodorants – entirely unnecessary, they can be HARMFUL.

Especially if they are scented. They also reinforce sexist ideas that female genitals are inherently nasty, and vaginal discharge is unnatural, undesirable and repulsive.

'The feminine hygiene industry is really shifting norms about what's normal – for profit. Many women feel anxious about something that's very normal and instead feel that they should all be smelling of rose petals or vanilla pods,' says Dr Bateson.

Dr Farrell also has clear views about 'hygiene' products. 'We don't need douches, we don't need extra things to put in our vagina or outside around our vulvas,' she says. 'We have millions and millions of bacteria in our vaginas that provide a cleaning process to make our vaginas healthy. We have pubic hair and the pubic hair has a function of protecting the vaginal entrance. And we also have our labia to provide protection around vaginas.

'The whole of the body has a very positive way of being and the concept of microbiomes, whether it be in the gut or in the vagina, is that it creates a healthy environment. Why do we want to change a healthy environment?'

Great question.

Your vaginal microbiome is an ecosystem made up of millions of microorganisms – including healthy bacteria and yeasts – that all work together. Each one of us has our own unique vaginal microbiome that is perfectly balanced when it's healthy. During puberty, when your oestrogen levels rise, a process begins that sees lactobacilli – the main bacteria in your microbiome – colonise your vagina. These healthy bacteria mix with cervical mucus and fluid from your vaginal walls to create your vaginal microbiome.

The lactobacilli help to keep your vaginal environment slightly acidic, which makes it difficult for harmful bacteria, yeast and viruses to survive. This reduces your chances of developing vaginal infections, such as yeast infections (thrush) and bacterial vaginosis. Your vaginal microbiome also plays a role in mucus production, which helps to rid your vagina of dead skin cells and other debris.

But this perfectly balanced environment can be disrupted by a bunch of things, including certain antibiotics, some lubricants, sexually transmitted infections and, you guessed it, FEMININE HYGIENE PRODUCTS.

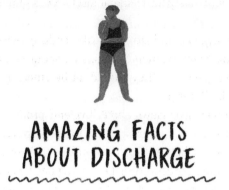

AMAZING FACTS ABOUT DISCHARGE

We want to share with you some of the other incredible things Dr Bateson told us about discharge and our marvellous self-cleaning vaginas.

Most women produce just under a teaspoon of discharge every day. Sometimes a bit more, sometimes less.

Sperm swim best in the mucus you secrete around ovulation. This is the time in your cycle when your discharge is stretchy and slippery, like egg white.

Your discharge can bleach your undies. Some of you may have noticed that your discharge strips colour from your undies; it's most obvious in black underwear, which ends up with an orange or yellow stain in the crotch. The cause? The slightly acidic nature of discharge.

I have always been so self-conscious about discharge. It wasn't until probably my mid-20s that I learnt what was normal and what wasn't and started to relax about it. That was until I became pregnant and my discharge started to BLEACH my underwear, and has done so ever since. It wasn't that it was a funny colour that washed off later, it was literally leaving those orangey bleach marks in my black underwear after they were washed. My calm was gone and I started to worry and become self-conscious, even hiding my bleached undies from my husband lest he comment. – **Amy**

Wear undies like your nanna's. The vagina likes to be in cool, airy surrounds; the yeast responsible for thrush, known as *Candida albicans*, thrives in a warm, moist environment. Go for comfy undies in a natural fabric (like cotton), and try to avoid any clothing that is too tight and damp – think sweaty activewear, wet swimmers or tight jeans. Wearing underwear at night also prevents the air from circulating around your vulva and increases your risk of thrush.

Stay away from scented panty liners. They can create an environment that upsets your vaginal microbiome and leads to infection. Dr Bateson says women often start to wear panty liners because they are worried about their discharge and how it smells, but wearing scented panty liners regularly can increase your chances of developing thrush or bacterial vaginosis – both of which will increase the amount of discharge you produce.

Not all itches are thrush. Thrush is one common cause of an itchy vulva, but it is not the only one. Bacterial vaginosis, dermatitis, worms and lichen sclerosus can all cause an itchy vulva. Go see your GP or health professional if you regularly get vulval itching.

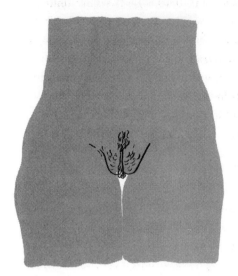 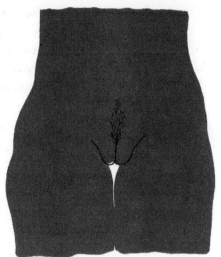

As Dr Farrell has pointed out, all vulvas are *unique*, much like our fingerprints. For instance, the most externally visible part of your vulva is your labia – and these can be smooth or wrinkled, dark or light, long or short. There's a fairly good chance yours are asymmetrical, as is the case with many parts of your body.

Unless you're having sex with women or in a line of work that takes you down there, you don't tend to appreciate the wide variety of vulvas that exist. Apart from your own, you see only a very specific type of vulva: the one that appears in the media – especially porn. This vulva isn't representative of *all* vulvas. It's a vulva that is smooth, with pubes neatly groomed or completely absent, and very symmetrical – where the labia minora are tucked neatly inside the labia majora. It's known as 'the clean slit'.

Many women are now feeling unhappy with the look of their own labia.

Dr Kang got a clue that labial appearance was becoming an issue for young women in the time before the Dolly Doctor column wrapped up in 2016. 'The question I started getting so much in recent years from Dolly Doctor, partly because of the fact that people remove their pubic hair and they get to see their labia more clearly, is the one about the inner labia protruding beyond the external labia. So there's a lot of anxiety about that, even though it's something like 20 or 30 per cent of women where that's the case.'

This dissatisfaction about our labial appearance is driving an increase in labiaplasty, the most common type of genital cosmetic surgery, which involves cutting back the labia minora (the inner lips of the vulva).

We don't know how common the procedure is in Australia as it's usually performed in private practice where surgeons are not required to report their data. But figures from the US Aesthetic Plastic Surgery National Databank show there was a 30 per cent increase in labiaplasty procedures between 2015 and 2019.

[Labiaplasty] is becoming a very popular procedure and many women get this done, but for some it has devastating consequences. Unfortunately, it's not as safe as the surgeons say. Nerve damage is a very high risk and as a result women suffer with severe sexual dysfunction, chronic debilitating pelvic pain, severe depression, pain with sex and total loss of sensation. I am one of these women and, unfortunately, there are many of us.

The surgeons downplay the risks, promoting it as a very safe procedure, while in fact they are cutting the pudendal branch in the labia which leads to horrific consequences. I can't even describe the nightmare my life has become since I had this done, and every single doctor I have seen told me that they are seeing more and more victims with the same complications.

This is a very embarrassing subject for women and most suffer in silence, not telling anyone. – **GINA**

Dr Gemma Sharp is a clinical psychologist and researcher who has looked at the reasons why women choose to have labiaplasty. She says women often don't like the appearance of their inner lips, or how they protrude beyond the outer lips. They have labiaplasty to get a smooth curve or a smooth surface.

Dr Sharp says there are two periods in our lives when we are most likely to be unhappy with our labia: in our late teens to 20s and then from our mid-30s to 50s, often after childbirth. A 2016 survey of Australian GPs on 'Female Genital Cosmetic Surgery' found that **girls as young as 10 were asking their doctors about labiaplasties and other genital cosmetic surgery**. Of the

443 GPs surveyed, 35 per cent said that girls under the age of 18 had asked them for genital cosmetic surgery. The big concern for young women having this surgery is that their labia haven't finished developing yet, and so they are at greater risk of scarring, loss of sensation and pain during intercourse.

'If we can start talking about labiaplasty and genital anatomy in general it can only really help young women and girls who are worried about this area,' says Dr Sharp.

'At least if they are concerned they might be able to reach out more easily, perhaps not go to the internet as their first port of call. Let's just start a conversation about these issues.'

✳ ✳ ✳

This expectation for a vulva to have smooth lines is partly due to trends in pornography, which overwhelmingly show vulvas where the labia minora are smaller than the labia majora, with both fairly symmetrical.

But even in non-porn content, our censorship laws don't help. Australian Classification Guidelines state that to legally stay within MA 15+ ratings, (which most mainstream film and TV entertainment aim to do): 'Realistic depictions of sexualised nudity should not be high in impact. Realistic depictions may contain discreet genital detail but there should be no genital emphasis.'

It's vague, but in classification laws that's been interpreted to mean that labia minora that protrude *beyond* the labia majora are considered too 'explicit' to be shown to mature audiences over the age of 15. Even though they are totally normal and common in the population. Translation? Some vulvas are more *pornographic* than others. So women's genitals are often airbrushed to that single crease to avoid an R 18+ classification.

On the other side of that rating, the R 18+ or X-rated side, the vulvas *also* tend to be a clean slit. This is the preferred look in most porn, in part because removing pubes and extra flesh makes it easier to see the 'action' clearly.

Even in non-sexual depictions, there's a genericness to how vulvas are represented. Research has found that women's magazines, when depicting the female pubic area in underwear, swimming costumes or activewear, tend to show it as a smooth curve or completely blank – like the plastic mound of a Barbie doll.

So we have laws, pornography and fashion all conspiring to tell the female population that when we look in the mirror, what we are seeing is NOT normal. This leads to fear, insecurity and dissatisfaction, or, to quote one's inner voice, *Eeeek! I'm not normal! I'm a freak!*

But what we must remember is that those beauty standards of what is 'normal' are being set by forces that DO NOT GIVE A DAMN about us.

Dr Bateson introduced us to an amazing resource called the Labia Library. As a response to the rising rates of cosmetic genital surgery, this online project was established to show women the extraordinary variety of labia.

She would also like to create something similar for discharge, not just for women but for their partners. 'I think a lot of the anxiety sometimes comes from their partners not recognising what's in this normal zone.'

Basically, it's time to stop caring about whether what's in our undies is normal – because you are normal! We are all normal! There is *no* normal! The spectrum of what is 'normal' is splendid and epic. And the spectrum of what we're shown is inhumanly narrow.

It's time to confidently and unreservedly accept that you have permission to be comfortable in your own body. To nourish it, care for it and do your best to understand it. To model acceptance to those you love and extend that compassion and acceptance to your global sisters and non-binary allies. To assuage any fears by sharing them with a doctor (more on page 190 about

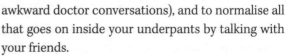

awkward doctor conversations), and to normalise all that goes on inside your underpants by talking with your friends.

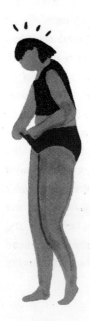

Remember, mates are an EXCELLENT resource. Every lady working on this book has had the experience of feeling slightly mortified about something that is going on with her body, only to find it's actually a normal thing once they talked about it with a trusted friend.

Trust and love? You give it to your friends. Now give it to yourself.

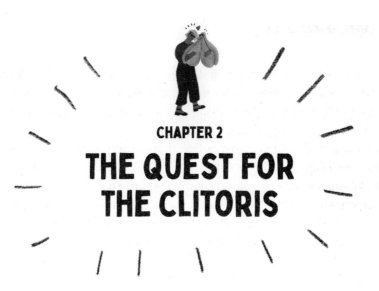

CHAPTER 2

THE QUEST FOR THE CLITORIS

The verdict is in and it's unanimous: most of us derive our sexual pleasure from the clitoris. If a woman wants to feel physical enjoyment from erotic experiences, then the best organ for the job is the clitoris. In fact, pleasure is its main purpose. Getting our partners to find it and apply the right amount of pressure, however, is a *whole other thing*.

But – and this is a pretty big *but* – it seems that many of us have trouble locating our OWN clitoris. Survey after survey suggests that plenty of us get quite lost when we go looking for it.

So, if the clitoris is the star of the female orgasm, why is she so underwritten?

For much of history, the clitoris – as a word, concept and body part – has been overlooked and ignored. Not only is it missing from medical texts, but it's also missing from sex education, from social media and from our MOUTHS.

Think about it – when was the last time you said the word 'clitoris' without feeling like you should lower your voice or check to make sure no-one would be offended by what you were saying? Did you cringe and steel yourself against the 'ugliness' of the word, like you were about to say 'phlegm' or 'queef'?

We're willing to bet you a butt plug that even if you got top marks in school sex ed, you didn't learn anything about the clitoris. It's almost like … *they didn't want us to know about it!*

But hang on – do you even really know about it now? Do you know the shape of your clitoris? What other body parts is it connected to? And, more importantly, do you know how to *find* it?

Ladies, we need to talk about the CLITORIS.

✳ ✳ ✳

The disdain for women's genitalia goes waaaay back and is embedded in the language that is used to describe our bodies. In the 1500s, when a French physician first dissected the clitoris, it was labeled 'membre honteux', which translates to 'shameful member'.

Dr Emily Nagoski is an author, self-confessed 'sex nerd' and virtuoso in women's pleasure. She says there was a view that women's genitals were tucked underneath their bodies because they were shameful, whereas men's genitals were front and centre. 'Why would [women's bits] be tucked away like that? Because god wanted women to be ashamed of their sexuality!'

PUDENDUM

Another name for the female genital package, which comes from pudēre meaning 'to be ashamed', which stems from the Latin pudenda meaning 'the shameful (parts)'.

Dr Nagoski says the clitoris was nowhere to be seen in the illustrations she saw in her school sex ed classes. 'Nowadays, if you're getting high-quality progressive sex education, you *might* get an illustration that has the little nub right at the top of the vulva'. (Refer back to the diagrams in chapter 1 if you need another refresh.)

She says there's a simple reason why the clitoris rarely rates a mention in class. 'Women's sexual pleasure doesn't really play a role in either male sexual pleasure or in reproduction. So why even bother talking about it?'

As for those awkward sex talks between parents and kids – pleasure is NOT the focus there. The first and only time Yumi heard her mum, Yoshiko, utter the word 'clitoris' was when she was a grown adult, recording the first episode of the podcast. Claudine has *still* never heard her mum say the word.

To be fair to our parents and sex ed teachers, people have NEVER been comfortable talking about female sexual pleasure and the importance of the clitoris.

Shocking fact?

We didn't even know exactly what the clitoris looked like until 1998, when a Melbourne woman published groundbreaking research.

Australia's first female urologist, Professor Helen O'Connell, is the legend responsible for leading the research team that fully mapped the anatomy of the clitoris.

When Professor O'Connell was training to be a surgeon back in the 1980s, the main med school textbook, *Last's Anatomy*, devoted pages to the penis, prostate and testes, their many nerves, and what happened to these body parts during an erection. 'You would have this very detailed description on the male anatomy and then you'd sort of have an addendum about the female bit.

'I was particularly eager to see whether or not these really big nerves were described properly. But all they had in terms of description was that "the female nerve follows the same pattern as the male nerve, but by comparison it's very small". That was it!

'I had to spend a fair bit of time with this book. Not only was there an absence of the anatomy of the clitoris, but some pretty pejorative language around female structures.'

Forgive us for defining a word you probably already knew, but it's worth drawing attention to the fact that the world often talks about women's bodies – in particular women's genitals and in particular the clitoris – in *pejorative* terms.

PEJORATIVE

Expressing contempt or disapproval.

The clitoris wasn't just given pejorative half-paragraphs in Professor O'Connell's textbooks. It's been pretty much ABSENT in academic anatomy texts, medical research or scientific journals throughout history.

For a long time the clit was considered the 'female equivalent of the penis', because of its structure, position and evolutionary origin. The word clitoris comes from the Greek word *kleitoris*, but it's not clear whether it was derived from *kleitys* (little hill), *kleiein* (to sheath) or *kleitoriazein* (to touch or titillate lasciviously). The term was coined by an Italian anatomist, Matteo Realdo Colombo. But his contemporary, the man known as the father of modern anatomy, Andreas Vesalius, had very little interest in the clitoris and pretty much denied its existence, saying that the clitoris did not exist in 'normal' healthy women.

When the clitoris did show up in research, the information lacked detail and contained inaccuracies – although we'd like to give a very honourable mention to Georg Ludwig Kobelt, a German anatomist who in the 1840s published intricate drawings and a comprehensive description of the female genitals, including the clitoris.

A real low point in academic appreciation of the clitoris came in 1948 when Dr Charles Mayo Goss deliberately ERASED it from the 25th edition of *Gray's Anatomy*, the bible of anatomy, of which he was the (male) editor.

Look, we don't know exactly why he made this decision. It could be that he accidentally lost the clitoris entry somewhere on the way to the printer. He might have forgotten. Maybe his low-level hum of disgust at this crucial organ grew so loud he was compelled to commit an act of academic vandalism so savage that modern women continue to experience the repercussions? We'll never know because, as (male) editor, he didn't have to explain his rationale.

One theory is that he subscribed to Freud's theories on sexuality, which were still quite popular at the time. Speaking of men who set back our understanding of the clitoris ... well, there are a few things to say about Sigmund Freud.

Freud was no fan of the clitoris. He theorised that women could only achieve sexual maturity when they had a vaginal orgasm while having penetrative sex with a man. In his 1905 work *Three Essays on the Theory of Sexuality*, he claimed that an inability to orgasm this way was a sign that a woman was 'frigid' and 'not a real woman'. His view was that reliance on clitoral stimulation for orgasm was evidence of 'immaturity'.

This idea may seem utterly ridiculous to us now, but it sparked a debate that has continued for more than 100 years. Those opposing the vaginal orgasm argument say penetration alone isn't going to bring most women to orgasm. Instead it's about direct stimulation of the clitoris by any means possible (finger, hand, tongue, sex toy ... whatever works for you). At various points in the last century, the pendulum has swung back and forth, with both sides of the debate pointing to published research that supports their view. It is worth noting that men were front and centre in the research that supports the superiority of the vaginal orgasm.

Where is the debate up to now? Well, technically it's still going. But without exception, every expert and woman we have spoken to agrees: if it's orgasms you're after, then focus on the clitoris. Some of us have wasted years of our sex lives feeling like failures because we couldn't orgasm vaginally when maybe we should have been having conversations with our partners about whether we need oral sex, certain types of clitoral touch or whether we'd just prefer to self-stimulate the clitoris during partnered sex. Sure, we can't blame Freud for all the problems with female sexuality, but his work certainly didn't help.

OK, where were we? That's right – no-one fully understood where the clitoris was, how it worked and what job it did. Even if you went looking for it in a medical book – the universal teaching tool on human bodies – it was like the clitoris ... did not exist.

It wasn't just the failings of anatomy textbooks that drove Professor O'Connell to change this. Early in her career, in the 80s and 90s, she would often see older women who didn't know their urethra from their vagina. Which is to say in layperson's terms: they thought they peed out of their vaginas. 'The lack of knowledge and disconnect between the owner and their body when it came to anything in the pelvis ... it was as though someone else did truly own it.'

During her training, Professor O'Connell and her peers were taught how to preserve a man's erectile function during prostate surgery. Yet no-one knew enough about the female anatomy to even *consider* preserving a woman's sexual function during procedures. 'In terms of surgery it's fair to say that the "normal" was male and anything that wasn't male was "other".'

If women were to get surgical treatments that weren't going to harm their sexual function, surgeons needed a better understanding of female anatomy. 'I was interested in knowing whether or not the same sort of nerves were present in women. And what sort of efforts had been made to define surgical pathways that would preserve the nerves if they were present.'

So she decided to do something about it ...

That something involved Professor O'Connell and her team spending hundreds of hours methodically dissecting the bodies of women, young and old, donated for medical research, to learn as much as possible about how the clitoris worked. They took photographs and did lab tests, so they could share this knowledge with other scientists and the world. 'Being able to dissect these noticeably large nerves and highlight their relationship to bony structures, to the vaginal wall, to the urethra, to the clitoris itself – it was an intrinsically worthwhile thing to do.'

The research published in 1998 included detailed information and photographs of the many dissections Professor O'Connell had performed. Then, in the early 2000s, she followed this up with MRIs that supported her earlier findings. 'I had to just keep on being true to what the findings were. I found myself on a journey that I didn't dream or expect.'

Did the pioneering professor realise she was changing the way the world understood this vital organ?

'To be perfectly honest, it was 1998. I was having a baby, I was running a medical practice. I was busy beyond belief. I didn't have much brain space to think of how this was all going to pan out from an impact standpoint.' (This probably sounds familiar, whether or not you're working on amazing anatomical discoveries.)

Professor O'Connell's work helped dispel centuries of misinformation about women's bodies and sexuality, and provided a solid foundation of evidence for everyone to work from.

She has come to appreciate how important this work is for those of us with a clitoris. 'It is very exciting if I've in any way helped people understand their bodies.'

I wanted to share why I love this podcast. It reminded me that when I was in first-year uni, at the age of flipping 19 (not that long ago – 2011), I learnt the full anatomy of the clitoris in a biology lecture given by a dude. He mentioned Professor Helen O'Connell's 'discovery' in 1998 and so many red flags entered my head. I was like: What the what – how have I gone through the mandatory state education system and no one has mentioned this? Mum, WTF? But also maybe you didn't know ... 1998, are you goddamn serious? I thought I lived in a progressive society – obviously a reality check. I had no idea I have this amazingly sized organ and only the tip of the iceberg – I've got some stuff to do! Thanks again for enlightening me (and all the women)! – **ANONYMOUS**

✳ ✳ ✳

We now know exactly what the clitoris looks like. And thank goodness we can actually show you an illustration of it, because it's hard to describe it in audio format. Creating a 'word picture' of what a clitoris looks like threw up some challenges for the podcast, and Yumi's solution was to compare it to a penguin.

Admittedly, it does look a bit like a penguin with its little flippers out. But instead of a round tummy, it's got two tummies hanging down like balls. And in a human body? All you can actually SEE of the penguin is its beak.

Imagine the clitoris as an iceberg: the only bits you can see or touch are the glans clitoris and clitoral hood (the penguin's beak). The remaining 90 per cent, which includes the crura and bulbs, is submerged, sitting inside the pelvis and wrapped around the bottom end of the labia, vagina and urethra. While the glans and hood are only a few millimetres long, the full clitoris can be up to 9 centimetres (about as long as a credit card).

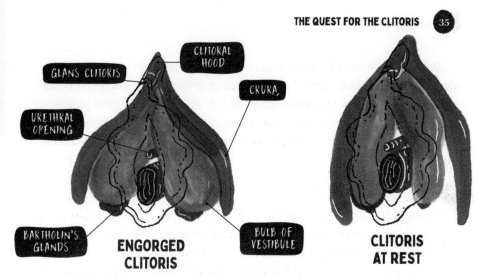

GLANS CLITORIS

CLITORAL HOOD

CRURA

URETHRAL OPENING

BARTHOLIN'S GLANDS

BULB OF VESTIBULE

ENGORGED CLITORIS

CLITORIS AT REST

Much of the clitoris is made up of erectile tissue that swells when you get aroused. So, much like a penis, your clitoris gets bigger when you're horny. And we're not just talking about the beak of the penguin getting bigger, we're talking about the whole thing – flippers, double tummies, ALL of the penguin! The bulbs of your clitoris swell and push into the walls of the vagina, which is ballooning out to make room for whatever is going in there, be it fingers, penis, dildo, cucumber, etc.

The clitoris is a high-quality sensory organ with up to 15,000 nerve endings. Its bulbs and crura are made of the same tissue as the penis. All these nerve endings are responsible for those tingly orgasmic sensations we experience throughout our pelvic area when we masturbate or have sex.

As for the controversial G-spot? The Grafenberg spot is supposed to be a few centimetres inside your vagina on the front wall, and some say it is a magical erogenous zone bringing orgasms galore ... if you can *find* it. But research co-authored by Professor O'Connell in 2016 found that it doesn't exist as an anatomical construct. The paper – 'The "G-Spot" is Not a Structure Evident on Macroscopic Anatomic Dissection of the Vaginal Wall' – gives it all away in the title. It also provides pretty compelling evidence that the reason this area can bring so much pleasure is because internal structures of the clitoris are on the other side of this spot on the vaginal wall, so it's clitoral tissue that is being stimulated.

The clitoris straddles the vaginal opening, so it can be engaged in certain positions during penetrative sex. And while extensive studies of female orgasms show that most women need clitoral stimulation to come, there will always be women who go their own way. Each of us needs to figure out which parts of our bodies give us pleasure.

A lot of us find the best way to reach orgasm during coupled sex is to stimulate the clitoris ourselves. Sexologists say the most common way for heterosexual women to reach orgasm during intercourse is through direct clitoral stimulation – often with our own fingers or hand. Yes, the male partner can sometimes have a crack, but we know the pressure we want, we know the kind of touch we prefer, we know the rhythm that works, and we know our fingernails are clean! Like they say: if you want a job done right, sometimes you gotta do it yourself. (There's a lot more on this in the chapter on the orgasm gap.)

Our favourite sex nerd Dr Nagoski has some sage advice for clitoris owners: 'The more we can make friends with our clitoris and welcome it precisely as it is, the more it's going to bring pleasure and joy into our lives.'

Pleasure and joy! Who doesn't want more of that?

Making new friends is always a bit awkward, but it can also be the beginning of something beautiful. If you'd like to make friends with your clitoris but feel as though you don't know where to start, Dr Nagoski says, 'The way we can change that is by learning to turn towards our bodies, look directly at our clitoris, touch our clitoris and explore it with curiosity instead of shame.'

Dr Nagoski is pretty clear on the first step to making friends with your clitoris.

> 'Go visit her. Get yourself a little hand mirror, take off your clothes and look at your vulva.'

Don't be alarmed if you feel uncomfortable about doing this. Dr Nagoski says she felt like she was confronting an enemy the first time she looked at herself in this way. She experienced a strong emotional reaction – but not because she was shocked by what she saw. 'I looked at my own genitals and I burst into tears, because it turned out to be nothing secret or scary or shameful or embarrassing at all. It was just a part of my body, just like all the other parts of my body.'

For Dr Nagoski this was a defining moment where she learnt that her body is the 'ultimate source of wisdom' on her sexuality – and she believes that's the case for all of us. 'Our bodies are already telling us what we need to know if we're willing to listen kindly and compassionately without fear.'

But given that approximately 90 per cent of your clitoris is *inside* your body, if you want to become besties with your clit, you will need to go a bit further than a peek in the mirror. You're going to need to get your hands involved in this exploration.

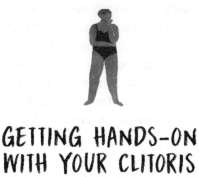

GETTING HANDS-ON WITH YOUR CLITORIS

Before you proceed, check in with yourself. Because self-consent is a real thing too. NOBODY has to do something they don't want to, even if it's obeying the voice in your own head saying, 'You *should*.'

You should do what you want.

You should also have clean hands and neat fingernails!

When you're exploring, be aware that the clitoris can be sensitive to touch, *not* sensitive to touch or *amazing* to touch at different times or stages of arousal.

OK? Good. Let's get started.

1. **Get comfortable.** Make sure you are in a space where you feel safe and comfortable. You want to take your time, so use any pillows or other props that are going to help you feel as relaxed as possible.

2. **Use lubricant if you want.** Dr Nagoski recommends using lube to reduce any friction that has the potential for tearing or pain. Lubricant will make sensations more pleasurable. 'Some people really like to use coconut oil. Others like to use a commercial lube. You can just use spit if you want to.' Go with what sounds good for you and your sheets.

3. **Start in your head.** You know that feeling when you're already in a sexy state of mind, a little bit turned on, and your partner tickles you and it feels nice? But if your partner tries to tickle you when you're in the middle of an argument, it's ... not so nice? Your clitoris is sort of the same. This is a long way of saying: sensations will not necessarily feel pleasurable and satisfying unless you're in a state of mind where it feels safe, welcoming and non-judgemental. 'Don't start with your hands. Start with your imagination,' says Dr Nagoski. 'Just say hello to your genitals from your brain. Think about them.'

4. **Notice the noise.** Notice the internal chatter going on in your head when you're feeling certain sensations – without any judgement. Dr Nagoski suggests asking yourself two questions: *What kind of emotions do you have when you touch your own body? And what sort of feelings do you have about your body and the sensations it's sending?* Allow yourself to explore what pleasure feels like.

5. **Work from the outside in.** When you are ready to touch yourself, start by gently touching the skin far away from your genitals. Touch your arms, legs, head or face. 'You want to notice what sensation feels like when you touch yourself,' says Dr Nagoski. Then when you are comfortable, and in your own time, move from the outer parts of your body towards the inner parts. Use your hands to touch along the insides of your thighs. Explore the area adjacent to the genitals – the mounds, the curves, the lines.

6. **Play with different sensations.** Our bodies are capable of so many different kinds of sensations, from light touch on the surface of the skin, to deep touch that pushes down into the muscles, to stretching sensations of tendons and muscles inside our bodies. Those sensations are all happening in different nerve endings in the skin itself. As you gradually move your way around your body and towards your genitals, give yourself time to experiment and to really feel each sensation.

7. **Breathe deeply.** Right down into your belly. Then imagine you can breathe down into your genitals – notice how that feels.

8. **Find your clitoris.** You've looked at your clitoris by now, so you know where it is. Now rely on touch to feel where it is. You might feel a rubbery-cord-type-thing underneath the skin right at the top where the labia divide – this is the shaft. Press down and feel the whole length of your clitoris. Feel the whole shape and size of it, knowing that it will change as you become increasingly aroused. These sensations may not necessarily feel super pleasurable or erotic, especially at the beginning, but this is an exploratory exercise (remember, you're just making friends).

9. **Notice how your clitoris changes.** As you begin touching your genitals, notice how it changes. Notice that the way it feels to touch your clitoris when your sexual arousal is at zero is not the same as when it's at eight or nine.

10. **Notice how your whole body changes.** Take a moment to notice how your whole body feels different. The tension in your muscles will feel different. The way your brain perceives a sensation is *really* different.

If making friends with your clit means really, really making each other feel good? At this point, you may be seized by an almost undeniable desire to continue stroking your new bestie. If orgasms have eluded you, there's no guarantee you can get them here, but it should still feel excellent. We've dedicated a whole chapter to addressing the orgasm gap, and masturbation is an essential part of training for pleasure. Turn to the end of this chapter for a beginner's guide.

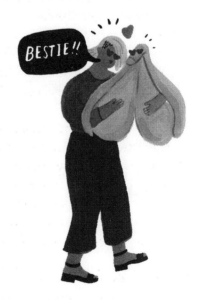

Comedian, actor and performer Tessa Waters was well into her 20s before she befriended her clitoris. The two had been briefly acquainted when Tessa was a child and had enjoyed rubbing herself against one of her favourite soft toys – a yellow five-pointed star pillow.

'I was sort of riding it like a horse and figuring out which point of the star was the most durable. I didn't actually orgasm, but I remember I was trying to be very, very quiet.'

Tessa also remembers feeling ashamed afterwards. 'I wasn't sure where this shame came from. My folks aren't the sort to make you feel that, and I didn't grow up with shame.' She just had the feeling that she'd done something wrong or forbidden.

'But there was also this sense of new strength that I had, and I didn't understand that either.'

Tessa's feelings of shame may strike a chord for many of us. From a young age, we're told not to touch ourselves, and when we do, our hands are slapped away or we're told we're dirty.

Dr Nagoski says these moments teach us that our bodies don't quite belong to us. Every time it happens it reinforces the message that 'there is a certain part of our body that is a source of disgust and horror. This one moment will accumulate with countless other similar moments until, by the time we get to adolescence, we can't articulate why, but we're barely aware of our genitals. We certainly don't feel like we could or should be touching our genitals.'

For Tessa these feelings meant 'I didn't masturbate again until I was in my 20s'. Yep, you read that right. Tessa didn't masturbate until she was in her 20s. For years she'd heard friends talk about clitoral orgasms and wondered why it hadn't happened to her.

She finally made friends with her clitoris when she was 29.

'When it finally happened and it was so amazing, I was relieved because I thought, "My body can do this."'

Then came sadness and anger, because she'd wasted time – and orgasms – thinking her body wasn't capable of experiencing that kind of sexual pleasure. 'I hadn't had [an orgasm] because I didn't know my body and I didn't feel empowered to ask my partner to help me discover my body.'

Soon after, Tessa started having sex with women and it was at this point her friendship with her clitoris, and with her whole body, really took off. What she learnt about pleasure was simple.

'It's about listening and it's about asking. It's much more about the whole pleasure, not just the coming at the end and the kind of triumphant-like, "Oh, well, I did really good!"'

These days, Tessa talks about the clitoris all the time. Actually, she doesn't just talk about it – she puts on her sequinned vulva shoulder pads and sings, dances and performs cabaret numbers about it with the Fringe Wives Club. Their show *Glittery Clittery: A Consensual Party* is all about combating misogyny and teaching audiences a thing or two about the female anatomy.

After every performance, audience members of all genders seek out Tessa and her bandmates to tell them how the show has changed their lives and their relationship with their clitoris.

I didn't know it was there.

I've never even said it aloud.

I feel like I'm allowed to be angry.

I'm allowed to ask for pleasure.

After one performance, Tessa's mum, Claire, was one of those people who found that everything had been cracked wide open.

'My husband and I were looking at one another, our jaws dropping, and saying, "How did we not know that?" We also both felt a bit sad that we didn't have the information ourselves to tell her as she was growing up.'

(Also sitting in the crowd at the show that night with Claire was none other than clitoris cartographer Professor O'Connell. When the crowd found out she was there, they started chanting: 'Melbourne's got the clit.' Yes, Melbourne's also got trams and terrible traffic, but for obvious reasons, the chant became a permanent part of Tessa's show.)

Watching Tessa's show made Claire reflect on what she hadn't shared with her daughter, as well as her own experience of being raised in a convent. She'd had about 10 minutes of sex education where she was taught about periods and reproduction ... and, well, that was it.

'Everything was just your bottom. You didn't know there were different parts. It was very, very confusing. I think it leaves you open to abuse and embarrassment and humiliation and mistakes.'

Claire thinks we're now in the middle of a sexuality revolution, one that started with the work of Professor O'Connell. And if she had her time over again, Claire would try to give her daughter Tessa a different understanding of her body. One that is based on simple and clear information, science and evidence, without the shame and guilt.

Claire also wanted to help change sex education in schools so she drew a 17-page illustrated guide to the male and female anatomies. 'If you don't know how your body works, how do you know what's normal when you go out there?'

Dr Nagoski has a fairly simple suggestion for how we overcome the clitoris taboo. 'The way we can conquer learnt fears or learnt disgust is by letting ourselves connect with that thing that we are afraid of or disgusted by.

'Clitorises come in so many different shapes and sizes and they are all healthy and normal, as long as they're not in pain. So, look at them! Have conversations like this about them! Learn to view them without that fear and instead just be like, "This is normal. Here's a clitoris. It's normal. Here's a different clitoris." It is a normal part of life.'

A BEGINNER'S GUIDE TO MASTURBATION

Yumi thought her school friends were cagey or private about masturbation and that's why they never talked about it. Later she realised a lot of them didn't talk about it because they didn't *do* it. Some didn't get started until well into adulthood.

If that's you too, it's pretty standard. In 2014, one of Australia's biggest ever sexual health surveys (the Second Australian Study of Sexual Health and Relationships) found that only ONE in FOUR women said they masturbated regularly – whereas half the blokes said they did. (Although we also need to allow for the fact that women might feel less comfortable admitting that they masturbate.)

If you're not masturbating regularly, you might not be a beginner at all, you might just be tired! It's hard to self-pleasure after a massive day of parenting or work stress. And while there are some heady life phases that are wild with wanking, there are quieter periods where the only kind of horny we feel is horny for doughnuts.

But experts agree that masturbation has a bunch of benefits that last way longer than your average orgasm. So, if you've made friends with your clitoris and are now ready to take the next step, here are some tips to get you started.

1. **Get your head in the game.** Like any kind of sex, masturbation is best if you're in the mood. What mentally turns you on? Watching good porn? Reading erotic literature? Fantasising about that hottie? (You know the one ... they never have to know.) Is it being on Day 14 of your menstrual cycle and getting a pay rise? There are everyday triggers that can send your hands diving into your underpants. Whatever they are, use them.

2. **Be safe.** Feeling like you have the freedom and privacy to explore is crucial. Lock the door, switch off phones, close laptops and make sure no-one is going to burst in.

3. **Clean hands, tidy nails.** You know this, but just sayin'.

4. **Get comfy.** Most people with a vulva like to spread it out. This might mean lying in bed, splaying your legs on the couch or arranging some sort of headrest in the bath. (A wank on the toilet is not as glamorous, but there are times when it'll do.)

5. **Touch the parts of yourself that want to be touched.** As we're going to learn in our chapter on the orgasm gap, our erogenous zones extend far beyond the clitoris and there are many ways you can touch yourself to build up your sense of pleasure. Remember: work from the outside in.

6. **No pressure!** In solo AND partnered sex, feeling pressure to orgasm can really be an orgasm killer. Since masturbation is just for you, there is no pressure to orgasm. You won't have failed if you don't. Relax and enjoy it.

7. **Stimulate your clitoris.** There are (literally) a million ways to do this: you can use your fingers, a pillow, a stuffed bear or a sex toy to caress, rub and stimulate your clitoris. Side-to-side, round-and-round motions are favoured. Mostly, they're repetitive and start off quite gently. Don't forget the bits on the inside. You can stimulate the internal parts of your clitoris by pressing on the shaft (the rubbery-cord-type-thing underneath the skin right at the top where the labia divide); by putting your thumbs, finger pads or the heels of your hand where the labia are connected to the body (your bulbs and crura are just below the skin surface); or from the inside by pressing the front vaginal wall of the vagina as you become aroused.

8. **Clench and release your pelvic muscles.** Imagine you're gripping something with your vagina, then letting it go. Repeat. This, combined with clitoral stimulation, contributes to the 'build' sensation as your pleasure increases.

9. **Pack up and go home.** Just kidding.

10. **Slightly increase pressure until explosions of pleasure make you want to stop.** This is called 'having an orgasm', and it's like fireworks from your fanny, laser-beam lightshows from your labia, an explosion of pussy butterflies – all the good things, all the good chemicals. And guess what? You did it all by yourself.

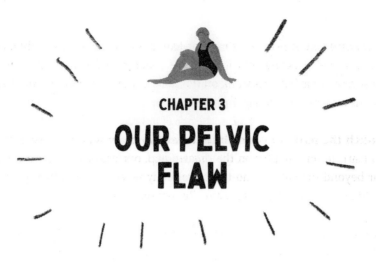

CHAPTER 3

OUR PELVIC FLAW

I f the charter of *Ladies, We Need To Talk* is to unpack taboos, then the need to talk about problems with the pelvic floor should be written into our constitution. It fits the criteria perfectly. Is it situated in the underpants region? Yes. Does it involve leaking or unruly female bodies? Yes. Do lots of us experience this thing? YES. And do we feel free to talk about it? NO.

When you look at the stats on prolapse and pelvic floor disorders (like these ones from the Continence Foundation of Australia), it's easy to see why listeners were begging for us to talk more about the pelvic floor.

- ★ Three quarters of those with any incontinence are women.
- ★ 1 in 3 women will experience some form of urinary incontinence.
- ★ 61 per cent of those who have given birth experience incontinence.
- ★ 50 per cent of those who have children will experience some degree of prolapse.
- ★ Pelvic floor issues can cause incontinence, pelvic pain and painful sex.

Prolapse – it's like a hidden secret and yet almost 50% of people who give birth will get one. Unfortunately I'm one of the unlucky ones who had one at the age of 36. Lateral avulsion (pelvic floor muscles torn off the bone, yet the birth itself was a great experience). There is no cure. Still struggling to come to terms with it four years later. – **LOUISE**

The stories come from women of all ages.

> I had a major pelvic organ prolapse after the birth of my first baby, who weighed in at over 4 kg, at the age of only 26 years. I saw my cervix popping out of me three days after my son was born. I was told to poke it back in and lie down. Literally – that was it. I was traumatised. I thought this only happened to old ladies. No-one talks about this! – **RACHAEL**

And even women who thought they knew more.

> I am a nurse and thought I was all over this but ... I had symptoms of pelvic organ prolapse and went and saw a gynae. The problem was that I didn't tell him ALL of the symptoms because I didn't realise that some of what I was dealing with on a daily basis were symptoms. I have now had several surgeries and am on the road to recovery. We really need to educate women about this as so many suffer urinary or faecal incontinence, prolapse, sexual difficulties, nerve pain, and that's just for starters. They are too embarrassed to talk about it. – **KATE**

We hear from women who work professionally on the pelvic floor, frustrated by the taboo that continues to surround pelvic floor problems.

> I am a 'pelvic floor and continence' physiotherapist and have been working with women for over 10 years now. On a daily basis I see women who have put off seeking help for far too long, either due to embarrassment of their symptoms, lack of awareness of the help available/where to seek it, or simply just because they feel that their symptoms are a 'normal' part of a woman's life that they 'cope with' because that's 'just the way it is'.
>
> Aside from my clinical practice, I find myself constantly being asked questions from family members, girlfriends, fellow mothers ... even my GP, about what it is I do, promptly followed by more hypothetical questions or queries about symptoms that their 'mothers' or 'friends' are

experiencing … Despite the increased conversation surrounding pelvic floor dysfunction across social media platforms and news publications, the taboo surrounding such issues is still very much present.
– ANNABELLE

There are a few things that regularly come up: 'I didn't know this could happen to me', 'No-one told me this could happen' and 'I want other women to know about the risks and how to avoid this situation'.

So, what we have is a common issue that affects many women – and we're not talking about it. Notice a trend here?

Ladies, we need to talk about our PELVIC FLOOR.

Dr Jenny King is a urogynaecologist at Westmead Hospital in Sydney and has spent decades working with women who've had prolapse, incontinence and other problems with their pelvic floor muscles.

She says there are a number of things that make women vulnerable to pelvic floor issues: genetics, having kids, hormonal changes around menopause, and a DESIGN FLAW. Our pelvic floor is the only thing between our internal pelvic organs – uterus, bladder and bowel – and the actual floor. It can usually keep everything in place when we are upright and walking around, but certain things (laughing, coughing, jumping or lifting) make its job harder.

When your pelvic floor is in tiptop condition it can handle extra pressure, but there are a bunch of things that weaken your pelvic floor over time.

'Heaps of us have a little bit of sagging on our vaginal walls, like we have sagging in our tummies. As soon as you start to get a little bit of stretching and sagging and changing in tissues, things will start to fall out and they fall out of that space of the vagina because they can,' says Dr King.

We found it pretty reassuring to talk to Dr King, especially about prolapse. She helped us to understand that being diagnosed with a prolapse does not mean you will have to become a recluse or have an operation or that there is nothing you can do.

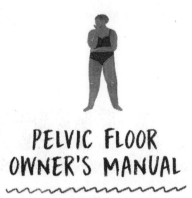

PELVIC FLOOR
OWNER'S MANUAL

Your pelvic floor is an underappreciated group of muscles, nerves and ligaments that attach to the base of your pelvis, pubic bone and tailbone. The main group of muscles involved are known as the levator muscles, and together they form a 'sling' that supports your bladder, bowel and uterus. Your pelvic floor has three openings: the vagina (leading to the uterus), urethra (leading to the bladder) and anus (leading to the bowel).

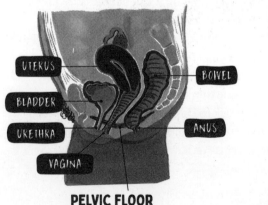

UTERUS
BLADDER
URETHRA
VAGINA
BOWEL
ANUS

PELVIC FLOOR

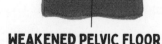

WEAKENED PELVIC FLOOR

What does your pelvic floor do? As well as keeping your pelvic organs – uterus, bowel and bladder – cupped and supported in their respective pelvic positions, your pelvic floor muscles help you to control when you pee and poo. They're also important for sexual function.

You know those muscles you squeeze in your vagina when you're having sex? That's them. The muscles you squeeze when you're doing your kegels? That's them too. You know when you're busting for the loo and can't find one but, instead of spraying pee everywhere like a malfunctioning lawn sprinkler, you huff and puff and bargain with god that you will absolutely promise to be a better person if you can just make it to the toilet this one time, AND YOU DO? Yep, that's your pelvic floor again, holding everything in.

Your pelvic floor muscles are absolute heroes in your life. They even help to stabilise your pelvis, hips and back. Your pelvic floor works really hard for you, so you should look after it!

What can go wrong with your pelvic floor? When your pelvic floor weakens or stretches it can cause incontinence, which involves losing control of your bladder or bowel and leaking either pee or poo. A weaker pelvic floor can also lead to reduced sensation in the vagina or to prolapse, where one of your pelvic organs moves out of place and pushes against the walls of your vagina or protrudes through the vagina.

Not every prolapse involves a uterus dangling from a vagina like a rogue abseiler! There are different types and degrees of prolapse, and sometimes you may not even know you have one as the changes will be internal. But do go see a pelvic floor physio or GP if you think you have a prolapse or if something doesn't seem right.

While we're focusing here on what happens with a weaker pelvic floor, it's also possible for your pelvic floor to be too tense. This can lead to painful sex and we're going to look at this in a lot more detail in chapter 12.

Why do things go wrong? There are some common causes for pelvic floor muscle weakness:

* pregnancy and childbirth (especially if the baby is over 4 kilograms or you pushed for a long time during delivery)
* being overweight
* straining when you poo

- ★ persistent heavy lifting
- ★ coughing (causing repetitive straining)
- ★ hormonal changes at menopause
- ★ growing older
- ★ genetics (some of us do have weaker connective tissue, which means that your pelvic floor muscles and ligaments are more prone to becoming weak)

How can you tell if your pelvic floor is struggling?

- ★ leaking pee when you cough, sneeze, laugh, jump or run
- ★ not reaching the toilet in time
- ★ frequently passing wind from either the anus or vagina (delightfully known as 'fanny farts') when you bend over or lift
- ★ reduced sensation in your vagina
- ★ a bulge at your vaginal opening
- ★ a feeling of heaviness in the vagina

What are the signs of prolapse?

- ★ feeling like you can't completely empty your bladder or bowel
- ★ a slow flow of pee
- ★ straining to pee or poo
- ★ leaking pee or poo
- ★ a feeling of fullness or pressure inside your vagina
- ★ a sensation of vaginal heaviness or dragging
- ★ a bulge or swelling felt in the vagina
- ★ lower backache
- ★ in severe cases, vaginal wall or cervix may protrude outside the vaginal entrance

Who should you see for help? If you have any symptoms or something doesn't seem right, head to your GP or a pelvic floor physiotherapist (we're going to be talking a lot about pelvic floor physios in this chapter). And if you don't feel satisfied with the information or answers you are getting, seek out a second opinion.

Lots of emails we get about prolapse come from women who have given birth vaginally.

Madeleine was 37, her third child was a couple of months old, and at her six-week check-up her obstetrician had said everything was fine. But a few days later Madeleine was sitting on the toilet doing a poo when she noticed something the size of a walnut bulging out of her vagina.

'It was very confronting and very upsetting and I think I may have texted my husband while he was at work saying, "Help! my vagina's falling out."'

She was shocked to discover she'd had a uterine prolapse. She'd been focused on the usual new mum list of worries – sleep, feeding, nipple care – but not on what was happening to her own body.

For months Madeleine visited a pelvic floor physiotherapist, who gave her exercises to help strengthen her pelvic floor, and they helped. But she will need to manage symptoms and maintain a strong pelvic floor for the rest of her life. While she's feeling pretty good these days, Madeleine struggles to use tampons and avoids certain exercises, like running or weightlifting. In good news, her sex life is still pretty great.

'I have felt demoralised and despairing at times. But there are treatments which do improve things, not fix it. It can certainly make your life a bit easier to manage.'

Madeleine wishes women, including health professionals, were more open with each other. 'I would love it if midwives and obstetricians talked, from the very outset, about how to mitigate risks, especially during birth, the positions you might be able to get into that might lessen the risk, and postnatal care.'

The word prolapse strikes fear into the heart of many women, but as we mentioned earlier there are degrees of prolapse. At one end of the spectrum, you may not even know that you have one.

Dr King says some women first learn they have a prolapse when they go for a Pap smear (also known as a cervical screening test). 'The GP will say, "Oh, this is bad, you've got a prolapse," but until then, the woman had no symptoms whatsoever.

'It's OK to sometimes leave it alone. If, say, you only leak when you do star jumps? Don't do star jumps! If you have a problem once a week when you're playing netball? Wear a pad. Not everything is a disaster.'

So what exactly is your GP or Dr King going to see when they examine someone with a prolapse? 'I part the labia on the outside, on the vulva, and I can see a softish little pink lump looking at me,' says Dr King. 'It may just come to the entrance [of the vagina], which is extremely common, or it can come past the entrance.'

Dr King says if you don't experience a birth injury and you look after your pelvic floor then your chances of having a prolapse or incontinence are significantly reduced. She certainly doesn't think that we should be opting for caesareans because we're worried about the impact of childbirth on our pelvic floor. 'It's partially protective for some women for a while, but you pay a big price for that caesarean section. There are complications. It is not so great for babies.

'Pregnancy probably explains 50 per cent of stress incontinence afterwards, and we know now from the big population studies that if you only had two children and both were by caesarean section, you would reduce your chances of moderate to severe stress incontinence by 5 to 10 per cent over someone who had had two vaginal deliveries, but only up to the age of 50.'

In other words? **Having a caesarean section instead of a vaginal birth will mean you are less likely to pee yourself while doing certain activities – but only by 5–10 per cent. Then after 50, age kicks in as the deciding factor.**

Dr King wishes more women understood this.

And while she wants to reassure us all that not all vaginal births lead to pelvic floor issues, she says that 'Childbirth does stretch vaginal tissue. I can tell if someone has had a vaginal delivery as opposed to a caesarean section, or no deliveries at all.'

As for the concern some women have that their vagina is too loose after childbirth? Well, Dr King says there isn't really anything you can do to restore that vaginal tissue, but pelvic floor exercises can help strengthen the muscles around the vaginal opening. 'All of that tension in the vagina that we use during intercourse is at the entrance. It's those pelvic floor muscles around the entrance. In intercourse the vagina walls in all women, particularly during orgasm, will blow out. There's no tightness against the penis higher up in the vagina. So [changes to the vaginal tissue higher up] really don't matter, if you can get your pelvic floor muscles working,' says Dr King.

So, don't freak out about things falling out of your vagina or your vagina being too loose – instead use that time and mental energy to focus on your pelvic floor exercises. (BTW we'll send you 50 bucks worth of incontinence pads if you've got this far into the chapter without squeezing and releasing.)

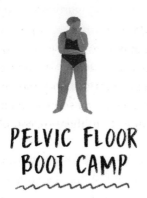

PELVIC FLOOR
BOOT CAMP

Like our fingerprints and vaginas, our pelvic floors are unique. So if you can, go talk to someone about your pelvic floor and what your body needs. A pelvic floor physiotherapist can help if you have any concerns about your pelvic floor and they can also make sure you're doing your exercises properly.

But if you want to have a go on your own, here's how pelvic floor physio Angela James says you can start. If you're thinking you don't need to do these because you haven't had kids or are nowhere near menopause, you are mistaken. It's recommended that we *all* do pelvic floor exercises every day.

1. **Find your pelvic floor muscles.** These exercises will help you find these muscle groups.

   ★ **Vaginal passage:** Insert two fingers into your vagina and try to squeeze them.
   ★ **Urethral passage (pee hole):** Visualise that you are peeing and try to stop or slow the flow. You can do this on the toilet while peeing, but you should only do it when you are trying to identify the muscles. Stopping your pee midstream is not an exercise.
   ★ **Anal passage:** Squeeze tightly and pretend you are trying to hold in a fart.

If you're finding it hard to identify these muscles, then it could be a sign your pelvic floor is weak and it's probably worth going to see a health professional.

2. **Get your technique right.** Don't waste your time doing your pelvic floor exercises the wrong way. Take the time to do them correctly. The following is a simple routine to get you started that can be done at any time.

★ **Get comfortable.** Either lie down on your back, sit down or, if you can, stand comfortably.

★ **Loosen up.** Imagine you are letting go of your pelvic floor muscles like you do when you pee or fart. Relax your tummy muscles too. Breathe in and out as you normally do.

★ **Squeeze and hold.** Keep breathing in and out with your tummy loose and then try to squeeze and hold in the pelvic floor muscles that you identified earlier. You might notice your tummy tighten a little below the belly button, but it shouldn't change above the belly button. You're only trying to gently lift and squeeze the pelvic floor muscles. If you can't feel your muscles contracting then change position.

★ **Relax.** Make sure you 'turn off' the muscles you have contracted. This is important as it allows them to recover from the previous contraction and prepare for the next. Many people try too hard and tighten external muscles – this shouldn't happen.

Once you are able to do these lying down or sitting, start trying to do them while standing. You need your pelvic floor to keep everything in place when you are standing, walking and moving around. If you're not sure you are getting these exercises right, go see a health professional. Doing pelvic floor muscle exercises the wrong way can make things worse.

3. **Up the reps.** Once you have mastered the art of squeezing your internal pelvic floor muscles while still breathing normally, try and repeat the exercise 10 times for each group.

When you are confident you are doing 10 repetitions without holding your breath or using external muscles, increase the amount of time you are holding each squeeze. It's a bit like working on your running from light jogging to doing sprints.

4. **Add some endurance.** Once you have mastered your sprints, you need to work on your endurance. Hold the squeezes for 10 seconds in a relaxed state, finish with 10 quick pulses to get quick fibres moving, then relax and let go. Repeat this 10 times.

   You should only switch to the endurance exercise if you are able to keep breathing during the 'sprints' and ensure your belly button is relaxed the whole time. The aim is to do the exercises in a *functional* way, so you also want to get to the point where you can do them standing up.

5. **Practise makes perfect.** When first starting with your pelvic floor exercises, do them often (up to six or seven times a day). Once you have mastered them, drop back to two to three times a day. Over time, strengthening these muscles with regular exercise can help prevent pelvic floor weakness and reduce symptoms of prolapse.

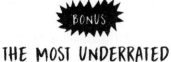

THE MOST UNDERRATED PLACES TO DO YOUR PELVIC FLOOR EXERCISES

The best place to do your pelvic floor exercises is anywhere that you will do them. Some women find it works well to get into the habit of doing them when they stop at traffic lights, when they are washing up or in the shower. Here's some other suggestions.

- ★ When a website says they'll send a code to your phone, in the time waiting for the notification.
- ★ When you hear the song 'drivers license' by Olivia Rodrigo, from the start of the build until the choir kicks in. That last release will feel EPIC.
- ★ When that wildly annoying person in your life talks to you. You can blink slowly, pretend to listen and picture your vag as a tattooed weightlifter doing bicep curls.

Many of us never even think about our pelvic floor – until we're exercising and suddenly it's the only thing you can think about. Pelvic floor physiotherapist Angela James is well aware that fear of leaking can hold people back from running and other fitness pursuits. 'The main message I'd like to get across is that exercise is so important for women and we would never hold a woman back from exercising.'

However, certain exercises – like running, skipping, lifting heavy weights and star jumps – put a lot of pressure on your pelvic floor. So if you have a prolapse or pelvic floor injury then before you do too much of these you should follow up with a pelvic floor physio or exercise physiologist who can make sure you're not doing more damage.

Even if you're only peeing yourself a *little* when you jump on the trampoline or go for a run, it's still worth going to see a pelvic floor physiotherapist. They can have a look at what is going on, check you are doing your exercises properly and work with you to develop a pelvic floor exercise plan that is going to work best for you.

They may also fit you with a pessary, which is just a fancy name for what is basically a really tough but very bendy bit of silicon that you put inside your vagina (as you would a tampon). It holds everything in place by supporting the internal structure of your vagina.

Pessaries come in a number of different shapes. The trick, Angela James says, is finding the right pessary for you.

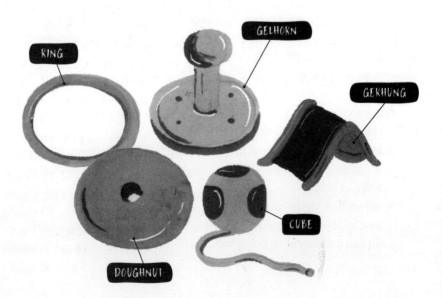

'Some women need to wear the pessary consistently because they have a pelvic organ prolapse and it's a really great non-surgical option for women.' But some of us will only need it when we're doing certain types of exercise, such as skipping or running or boot camp.

'If you have a dodgy knee ligament but you love playing touch footy, we get you to wear a knee guard. It's the same thing if you've got a slightly dodgy pelvic floor muscle but you love skipping – we get you to wear a pessary to make sure the area is supported.'

After Yumi spoke to Angela James for an episode of *Ladies, We Need To Talk*, she quietly made an appointment to see her. During the interview James had mentioned that if you've had a few babies (Yumi has had four), pelvic floor physio shouldn't be seen as a luxury – it's just maintenance, like going to the dentist!

Yumi's check-up was as you'd expect – one of those what you might call 'The Undies Are Gonna Come Off' specialist appointments. A pessary was also recommended, and later fitted, and straightaway Yumi felt like, 'Yep, this is good. I've done the right thing.'

The pessary took away the feeling of heaviness she was having around the opening of her vagina. Yumi says it's hard to explain how the pessary works, but imagine your organs bearing down from above trying to escape out your vagina – except now there's this robust object in the way, keeping the organs from heading south.

Most weeks Yumi will go on a 10-kilometre run at least twice and she now doesn't even have to *think* about her pelvic floor when she's exercising.

Angela James told Yumi that the accountability of having regular check-ups of your pelvic floor is incredibly useful for helping women stay on track with exercises and general pelvic floor health. That really stuck with Yumi. After that first visit, she went back for six-monthly check-ups and now she goes once a year.

So, what exactly should you expect from a pelvic physio appointment?

There are specialist clinics that just focus on pelvic floors, and the staff and physios are often all women. These are spaces where you should feel very safe and understood. No one is going to be squealing in disgust at your situation.

When it's your turn to see the specialist, you'll usually sit down and talk about your reason for being there that day, just like a regular GP appointment.

Questions will probably cover: urinary continence and bowel function; how many, if any, babies you have carried and what the births were like; your sex life, including whether you find sex painful; if you feel any symptoms of prolapse (heaviness, lump or bulging inside the vagina or rectum); your exercise habits (including whether you already do pelvic floor strengthening exercises); what concerns you the most, and whether you have been to a pelvic floor physio before (they're asking if you know what to expect).

Then comes the examination. This is a pretty standard undies-off procedure. She will ask you to lie down on your back in a situation very much like when you're getting a Pap smear or an IUD. She will probably cover your lower half so you don't feel exposed, then talk you through what she's doing as she does it.

This includes doing a visual check of the outside area of your vulva, then using a gloved hand to stick two fingers inside your vagina and asking you to contract your muscles, cough, bear down and try to use other muscles to squeeze on her fingers. She also uses a device to measure the strength of your muscles so that there's a reference next time you come back – you can check if things have improved, worsened or stayed the same.

If your main problem is rectal incontinence, there will be the same sort of questions, checking and clenching, just with a (gloved) finger up your butt.

After that? It's undies back on time!

Sometimes your physio will check your posture (sitting and standing) and will want to weigh you. This can all be done from the comfort and safety of your undies. And she may ask you to keep a bladder diary.

This is now your chance to ask her a bunch of questions too, like:

★ What's going on?
★ Does it look OK?
★ If I don't do anything, will it get worse or better?
★ Is this something you see a lot?
★ What can I do to help myself?
★ Can I improve?

Aside from doing your pelvic floor exercises or using a pessary, the only other treatment option for prolapse or incontinence is surgery. But that's something Dr King says isn't necessary unless your pelvic floor symptoms are affecting your quality of life – that is, 'not potentially affecting your quality of life in the future, but now. So it may be blocking the bladder, stopping it from emptying, making it difficult to empty the bowel, coming outside and rubbing, and perhaps bleeding, on your underwear.'

Dr King wishes we'd all be a bit more willing to speak up when something goes wrong with our bodies.

'If you get that leaking with the star jumps at the gym, if you notice something bulging down there, it is worth having it seen to. You may save yourself a lot of problems later on and you'll keep your body as good as it can be. Please pluck up the courage and go and see your GP.'

We would love all women to stop feeling ashamed and embarrassed when it comes to our pelvic floor. In fact, all of the women who contacted us want that too. They want women to stop feeling ashamed or embarrassed about incontinence, prolapse and other pelvic floor issues and for there to be more honest conversation around these challenges.

As Madeleine says, 'Prolapse is a horrible word, like your body is lapsed. It's made some kind of mistake, some major error, but you haven't done anything wrong. You're not responsible for it.'

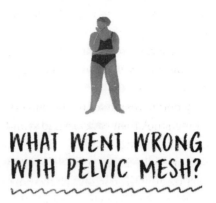

WHAT WENT WRONG WITH PELVIC MESH?

'A lot of the stories were very similar. They had no options. They had no options in terms of getting the mesh taken out, and in a lot of cases they just had to live with it, which is pretty rough when you are just told to live with debilitating pain every day.'

Sophie Scott has been the ABC's medical reporter for more than two decades, but she'll never forget her conversations with women whose lives were devastated after having pelvic mesh implanted.

Scott says women contacted her to share their stories because they were living with debilitating pain that was taking a terrible toll on their mental health, lives and relationships – and no-one would listen to them.

When they tried to talk to their doctors they were told what they were experiencing was 'all in their head' or the pain was 'just part of the recovery process'. These were sometimes doctors who they had trusted and known for a very long time.

Pelvic mesh or transvaginal mesh products, including slings, tapes and ribbons, are synthetic net-like substances used to support weakened organs and help strengthen internal tissue. When it first came on the market, pelvic mesh was heavily marketed to doctors as a simple and quick surgical solution for urinary incontinence. It was then offered as an option for prolapse. It wasn't the only surgical treatment for these conditions, but it was one that didn't require the same level of surgical expertise as other treatments.

It's been estimated that more than 150,000 women in Australia had pelvic mesh inserted, and for many of these women it improved their symptoms and caused no side effects. But a significant number knew something wasn't right when they began to experience symptoms such as irregular vaginal bleeding, pelvic pain, discomfort during sex, bladder and bowel problems, or pain in the leg, abdomen or butt.

Sometimes these symptoms came soon after surgery, but for others it took years. When these women took their concern and symptoms to their doctors, they were told it couldn't be the mesh and that they just needed to give things a chance to settle. But rarely did things 'settle'; often they got worse.

'These women were really at the end of their rope in terms of trying to seek help,' says Scott. 'It was only really when they got together that they realised they had this commonality of experience – in terms of the pain they were suffering, not being listened to by their doctors, really poor quality of life and no-one else to turn to.'

The women's stories were finally heard in a 2017 Senate inquiry. Thousands of Australian women shared their experiences of the 'devastating complications' from transvaginal mesh implants and how they had been 'ignored' and 'treated appallingly' by their doctors and regulatory bodies. Many women said that they were not made aware that there were risks associated with pelvic mesh, and that if these had been properly explained to them then they may have made different decisions.

The final report from the Senate's inquiry was damning of medical professionals and regulatory processes. After it was handed down, doctors' groups and the federal government apologised, the mesh was banned as a treatment for prolapse and the women were awarded damages by the courts.

Scott says the women she spoke to all wanted the same thing from telling their story. 'They knew it was too late for them, but they wanted to make sure that other women knew the risks of this pelvic mesh implants and they also wanted to make sure that doctors knew that they couldn't just ignore their patients.'

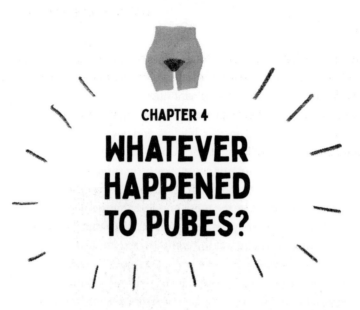

CHAPTER 4

WHATEVER HAPPENED TO PUBES?

When it came to talking pubic hair, *Ladies, We Need To Talk* was looking for someone to interview who had direct, daily access to women with their pants off. Specifically, someone who looked at women's vulvas – and that someone could *not* be a hair removal technician.

Enter Dr Talat Uppal. Dr Uppal is a Sydney-based gynaecologist and obstetrician, who looks at vulvas most days. From the full Brazilian to the full bush; from heart shapes, maps of Tassie and landing strips to vajazzled vulvas with piercings and dye – when it comes to pubic hair, Dr Uppal has pretty much seen it all. A veritable vulva spectacular!

But, mostly? Dr Uppal is seeing a lot LESS pubic hair.

Every single day at her clinic, a client will apologise for the state of their vulva. 'It's some sort of apology for either the smell or the hair or ... what they perceive as less hygiene than they would have liked,' says Dr Uppal.

Her response is always the same. 'Don't apologise. You absolutely don't need to think about this when you come to see us. No-one is judging and no-one has any preconceived ideas of what normal is. Normal is what is normal for you. And our role is just to look after you.'

When people come to be examined by Dr Uppal, it's for a gynaecological or obstetric issue – pelvic pain, heavy period bleeding, ovarian cysts, pregnancy – and yet there they are, apologising for the state of their pubes. 'I don't know whether it is perceived as something you are meant to do, like brushing your teeth when you're going to see the dentist. But we're certainly not expecting any "work" before you come to see us.'

Pubic hair hasn't just disappeared from Dr Uppal's clinic. It has disappeared *everywhere*.

Ladies, we need to talk about our PUBES.

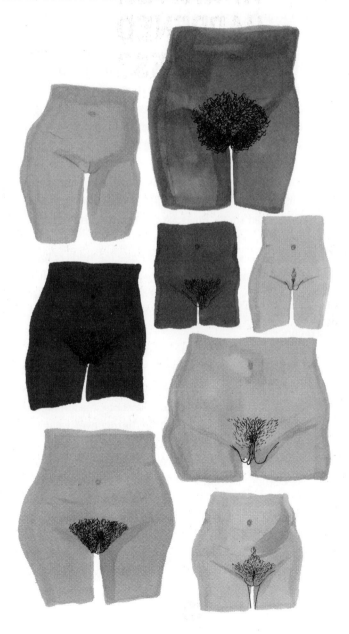

✳ ✳ ✳

When was the last time you saw a pube? At the beach? In pop culture? In a public change room? Over at your friend's place, lurking inside her famous lasagne?

These days most of us do some form of pubic hair grooming. Even if you *aren't* deforesting your native bush, you're still likely doing regular maintenance to keep the edges tidy.

There's not a huge amount of research into pubic hair removal practices, but one regularly cited US study found that **60 per cent of women got rid of all their pubic hair at some point in their lives**, and close to 85 per cent groomed. While this study (from *JAMA Dermatology* in 2016) suggests it is 'younger, white, college-educated and well-paid women' who are most likely to be grooming their pubes, it is still something that cuts across age, race and education.

Across cultures, hair removal has a long history. It turns out that tweezing and plucking is as ageless as wagging school on Cross Country days, except that people in the past used shells, flints, pumice stones and bamboo – along with fingers, of course – to get those hairs out.

Over the years, less successful and more extreme methods of hair removal have come and gone. For example, at one stage people used thallium – a type of rat poison – as a depilatory or hair removal cream (ouch)! In the early 1900s, X-rays zapped hairs away painlessly but had the nasty side effect of causing radiation-related cancers.

For some cultures, hair removal hasn't been such a big thing.

In Japan, where Yumi's ancestors are from, women leave their thatches of pubic hair intact. (You can check for yourself if you ever go to one of the public baths in Japan.) Yumi's Japanese friend Itsuko says one reason Japanese girls don't go for pubic hair removal is because they hardly ever wear swimwear. In Japan as well as China, to remove the hair of the body is seen as hurting it – and as our skin and hair is received from our parents, we should not presume to disrespect them by removing it. (That said, armpit hair removal has become mainstream in Japan, but less so in China.) In parts of Africa, thick and luxuriant pubic hair is seen as a mark of female beauty.

In Australia, where beach and surf culture is a massive influence on even the most land-locked non-swimmer, managing and removing pubic hair really started to take off after the bikini arrived in the 1940s, mostly to take care of any 'koala paws'.

I'm in my late 40s and I've never had a Brazilian, although I have plucked, trimmed and used depilatory creams to stop the 'koala paws' escaping my swimwear. – **JOANNE**

The eradication of the pube got serious in the late 90s when the Brazilian wax became popular. Brought to the US by the J Sisters at their New York salon in the 80s, the Brazilian removes all the hair from your mons pubis, labia and pubic area – as well as any from your butt crack. Basically, it ALL comes off.

The first time I got a 'full' Brazilian wax, I had not been told that they did the bum area as well. LET ME TELL YOU, my eyes went so wide they were visible from outer space! – **SARAH**

While Brazilians started off as a specialised waxing treatment offered by salons, people soon began to DIY with razors or wax at home. Nowadays, many women nuke their pubes away forever with permanent laser treatments, resulting in a generation of women date-stamped by irreversible pube removal.

Diane is a beautician who says she's 'seen it all' in her 20 years in the industry. 'Laser and IPL have changed the industry – because trends change and fashion changes but permanent hair removal is forever. It's not very regulated and I've seen people get burnt from it, including myself!'

As a 53-year-old German who has lived in Brazil, the UK, the US and Oz, I've been exposed to a lot of different cultural perceptions regarding pubes.

In the late 80s in Germany, ALL the women had pubes and hairy legs! Only a Chilean friend of mine at the time said she couldn't imagine it, because her mum had brought her up to shave her armpits and legs, as well as trimming the pubes.

When I moved to Brazil in 1991, my then new husband said he didn't mind my hairy legs, armpits and pubes (I'm not very hairy though). But he did warn me that ALL the women had shaved legs, armpits and trimmed pubes. After a week or two at the beach, I felt like a gorilla (wearing a turtleneck sweater because of my European-sized bikini)! I started shaving and trimming. In the 90s the customary depilation was quite thorough because of the tiny bikini briefs or thongs – but never removed everything!

I remember the feeling of total weirdness to remove my hair – because no-one else did where I came from! Now I can't see myself ever having hairy armpits or legs (or pubes showing) because of the same reason. So, to me, it's quite clear that the whole thing about having or not having body hair is purely cultural and aesthetic – nothing to do with hygiene or individual attraction. – **SILKE**

Why are we doing all this shaving, plucking, waxing and lasering?

Comedian and finance manager Christina Zheng knows exactly why she gets rid of her pubes. 'It makes me feel clean, confident and ready for anything. I think the feeling after a fresh wax is just incomparable. I feel like I can tackle anything, like one of those girls in the tampon commercials.'

Christina reckons her regular Brazilian gives her so much more confidence that she chose to have one right before she gave birth. 'I remember going to a birthing class at the hospital and watching a video, and you could tell it was made in the 70s. Everyone in the class audibly gasped at the sight of the magnificent bush, but we agreed it was also a huge visual obstruction. I just wanted to make sure the obstetrician had a clear line of sight.

'It was funny, because my baby came out with a full head of hair as she's half Lebanese. And when I was crowning, the nurse handed me a mirror. I was so heavily drugged and I freaked out because I thought my pubes had grown back in three days.'

Dr Hannah McCann is a senior lecturer at the University of Melbourne, researching beauty culture. She says, 'Consistently, surveys of women around why they remove body hair [show] an association with being hygienic, and being clean and, with specifically pubic hair, hygiene and sexual attractiveness. Paradoxically, altering your body from what it would be naturally is seen as a way of achieving "normality".'

That oft-cited US study also looked at motivation for removing pubic hair. It's probably not a surprise to hear that many of us groom our pubes when we plan on having sex or going on holiday. No surprises that we like to groom because we think our partners like it and that it makes our genitals more attractive. But **the most common motivation women give for grooming is HYGIENE**.

So, let's talk about hygiene.

Humans have evolved to have pubic hair – it protects the vulva. Think of pubes as being like the eyelashes of your vulva. As we discussed in chapter 1, your vagina is an amazing self-cleaning structure and your pubic hair plays a role in this. Dr Uppal says pubic hair creates a physical barrier that 'traps either debris, pathogens or bacteria or foreign material' and can reduce your chances of developing vaginal infections.

Your pubes are also a buffer – think about how your undies sit away from your skin when you have pubic hair. This can help with airflow and stop fabric rubbing against the very sensitive skin of your vulva. Pubes also seem to keep your undies cleaner! BONUS.

That so many of us think of pubic hair as being unhygienic – when its very role is to help keep the vulva clean – is a bit confounding.

Dr McCann thinks that 'scientific' positioning in beauty advertising may have something to do with it: 'it's about achieving "hygiene" and "cleanliness" while positioning itself as scientifically advanced. There's always the invention of new machines that can remove hair. Laser! Wax! They emphasise the relationship between science and beauty.'

Even though many of us remove pubic hair because it makes for a 'smoother' sexual experience, pubic hair is actually sometimes referred to as 'dry lubricant'. Basically, it's easier to rub hair against hair than it is to rub skin against skin.

Dr Uppal explains, 'It minimises the risk of trauma because it's a layer and is not exposing raw skin on raw skin. It's a sort of mechanical barrier.'

There's also been debate about whether the pubic hair barrier protects against sexually transmitted infections. Some studies have found that those who remove their pubes are more at risk of certain STIs, while other studies have found no connection between the two things.

Researchers have never been able to find a clear biological reason for why pubic hair grooming might cause STIs. One theory for the research findings is that those more likely to groom their pubic hair may also be more likely to have multiple sexual partners. It's also worth noting that some of the studies involved self-reporting, which can be unreliable.

To further confuse things, a paper from 2019 found *no* link between removing pubic hair and an increased risk of STIs. (What was really interesting about this paper, published in the US journal *PLOS ONE*, is that more than

98 per cent of the women involved in the study groomed their pubic hair, but they were all English-speaking uni students.)

So, what's the take-home message?

1. Research is complicated – don't just read the headline.
2. Practise safe sex – don't leave it up to your pubic hair to protect you from STIs.

The biggest health issue related to pubic hair is the INJURIES that occur when we're getting rid of it. Not what you expected, huh?

There's a long list of injuries associated with pubic hair removal. Some of these happen during the process, such as cuts or bruises, and some injuries arrive a little later, such as ingrown hairs, infections, rashes, and even sepsis (a very serious condition caused by infection).

Diane says, as a beautician, she's seen a lot of clients trying to DIY during COVID. 'They stop after one side because they can't follow through, so they have half a Brazilian. It's easy to pull a big bruise on yourself if you don't know what you're doing.'

A 2017 US study on the 'Prevalence of Pubic Hair Grooming–Related Injuries' found that **about one-quarter of those who groom their pubic hair will be injured while they do it**, and it's women who are more likely to be injured than men. To avoid this, we suggest you read on.

You mentioned some of the consequences of shaving, waxing and laser, but failed to mention the risk for darker-skinned WoC of post-inflammatory hyperpigmentation (PIH). I gave up shaving as often because, after lots of research, I realised the increasing darkness downstairs actually gets worse with regular shaving. I told all my siblings and cousins, and they also stopped doing it as often after finding out!

Darker skin tones get left out of new beauty treatments and conversations a lot! Most of what I know, I find out myself. Many WoC don't even talk about it or mention it! My PoC dermatologist never even told me properly about PIH until I asked her because she's so used to catering to white-relevant information. So, there are added considerations if you have dark skin, not to mention the extra pressure and cost for hairier women to keep up with hairless beauty standards as compared to thinner- and fairer-haired women. – **ROSANNE**

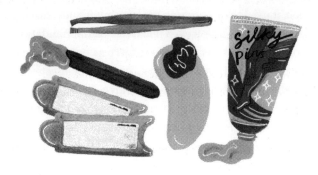

YOUR SAFE PUBES REMOVAL GUIDE

You know how common it is to remove pubes, and that doing it wrong can cause injuries? Well, it's still surprisingly hard to find any guidelines on how to turn your fuzzy triangle into a little snatch of velcro. So, we've done the hard work for you. You're welcome!

SHAVING

- ★ **Pros:** Cheap, quick, equipment is easy to find and you can DIY (or with a partner).
- ★ **Cons:** Hair grows back quickly, high risk of cuts and scraping, microabrasions (removal of minute amounts of skin) can foster bacteria, risk of reaction and ingrown hairs, and the itch of regrowth is like a colony of murderous ants taking up residence under your skin.
- ★ **Getting it right:** Always use a new razor so it's both sharp and uncontaminated. Wet and lubricate the area, hold the skin tight and shave in the direction your hair is growing. Oh, and don't shave over a scab.
- ★ **Horror story:** 'It's actually the regrowth of hairs that become ingrown and then they form abscesses,' says Dr Uppal. 'I've had to take patients to theatre to drain these sorts of injuries because they've caused an infection and there's a collection of pus there.'

★ **Special note:** Don't shave before you give birth vaginally or via caesarean; it used to be common practice but it's now discouraged (the World Health Organization even released a recommendation on it). 'It's better for us to clip it just prior to surgery as opposed to you shaving any time prior to that,' says Dr Uppal. Your risk of infection increases if you have shaved, especially in the pubic area. 'That area is not a flat line so it is quite possible to create microabrasions, or it's a fragile skin that can have cuts which then predisposes it to an infection.'

WAXING

★ **Pros:** Longer lasting, very smooth finish, significantly less itchy when growing back – and the pain of the hair being torn out wakes you up like a slap in the face if you're feeling sluggish.

★ **Cons:** It hurts, can be expensive if you get it done at a salon, is hell messy if you DIY, plus there's risks of burns, ingrown hairs and other injuries. And you need to snap the wax off in the right way or you can bruise your skin.

★ **Getting it right:** If you DIY, make sure everything you are using is clean, make sure the wax isn't too hot, don't share any equipment with anyone else, and avoid double-dipping of used spatulas into the wax.

★ **Horror story:** Dr Uppal says we need to be careful with waxing as we get older. 'With older women, because of the low oestrogen stage, your skin might be a bit more fragile than it used to be. So, with waxing, I've seen removal of the top epidermal layer of the skin, exposing the underneath – that has not been pleasant.'

★ **Sugar waxing:** This low-enviro-impact version involves making a dough-like 'wax' out of sugar and water, using your fingers to spread it in small patches over the area you want to remove hair from, then snapping it away off the skin. It's got similar cons to standard DIY waxing (plus it's more time-consuming) BUT it's cheaper, not horrendous for the environment, and it smells kind of like toffee.

CREAMS (ALSO KNOWN AS DEPILATORIES)

★ **Pros:** Cheap and easy to do at home, creams come in all delivery systems, from sprays to roll-ons to your standard tube or jar of cream. It's quick (you apply the cream then leave it on for 3–10 minutes), no pain unless there is an allergic reaction, and most creams no longer smell like Satan's farts.

★ **Cons:** can irritate the skin causing anything from mild irritation to blisters and burns, hair is removed only to skin level so grows back within days. And some brands still smell like Satan's farts.

★ **Horror story:** 'I was so impressed with how easy depilatory cream was on my legs that I decided I'd go a bit higher but accidentally used Deep Heat cream instead!' We can feel the burn.

LASER

★ **Pros:** It's permanent, so after a certain number of treatments you never have to think about it again.

★ **Cons:** It's permanent. It's also expensive, only works on hair that is darker than skin tone (greys and blonde hairs cannot be successfully removed), can result in permanent pigmentation or scarring or injury, and hair can grow back requiring follow-up treatments.

★ **Getting it right:** Space out the treatments, be aware of the risk factors and make sure you have the right treatment modality for you. Avoid sunlight for three days after treatment.

★ **Horror story:** 'I was always mindful to take a shower before having an "X-rated laser" session because I didn't want the therapist to have to deal with smells and discharge. One time I was in there, having showered, the laser zapped one tiny spot on my anus that must have had a single molecule of poo clinging to it, and the room filled with the smell of barbecued faeces.'

ELECTROLYSIS

★ **Pros:** Pretty quick (between 15 minutes and an hour), with less heat and fewer side effects than laser (as electrolysis uses radio waves), and recognised by the US Food and Drug Administration as the only permanent method of hair removal.

★ **Cons:** Not cheap and multiple sessions are required, and can result in redness.

★ **Getting it right:** Forget about trying it at home. Get an accredited technician to do it, preferably someone who has experience with your skin type. Should not be used in tandem with laser.

OK, if we can accept that pubes are actually good for us, and the whole 'smoother' illusion that goes with hairless sex is a myth, then why is it so hard to ignore that feeling of *Oh my god, they'll think I'm a freak if I have a free-range bush*?

Tradition and expectation play a big part. 'There are some ethnicities that have thicker, bushier hair than others,' says Dr Uppal. 'Pubic hair doesn't necessarily always match up with the hair on women's heads, whereas there might be that perception that it has to be exactly the same texture or colour or thickness.'

For many young women, what their friends are doing is the most powerful influence. 'I'm aware of patients that are basically grooming themselves from the beginning of puberty. I think that's a group in which peer pressure is very important,' says Dr Uppal. These young women are in social media groups sharing personal stories and information about hair removal from a range of sources. 'But many times when girls share their experiences with their friends, they don't share the negative part of hair removal,' Dr Uppal adds. 'So there's a potential to glamorise this while not being mindful of the price tag of some of the choices we make.'

Dr Uppal says we need to make sure we're not just skimming the surface when it comes to hair removal. 'It's not just a social removal of hair. There might be other deeper and important issues around self-esteem or self-objectification.'

Dr McCann asks us to consider again what we see in the advertising, the media and in pop culture. 'Products promoting removal of body hair are sold as a way of controlling your body. A hairy body is seen as out of control, masculine, and unruly ... The way that advertising is working now is really different from a print magazine ad. You have influencers EMBODYING the look – so their persona is the thing that you're trying to achieve.

'You can say all these things about beauty as identity, curating the self, etc. But the beauty industry has an interest in you wanting to remove hair. It can't exist without the desire for you to change your body.'

Of course, we still have choice and agency in these situations. 'Women know a lot about these pressures and are aware of them – you can't discount women's complex knowledge and engagement with these things.'

Interestingly, pubes became endangered at the same time that porn became as accessible as the phones in our pockets. Unless it's a kink, we don't see pubes in porn and this creates an expectation that pubes have no place in hot sex.

Back in the olden days (when our parents still had sex), a fully hairless mons pubis as seen in porn used to be salacious and risqué. It was considered titillating and naughty and it was *different* from what Mum and Dad saw at home in the bedroom.

But as porn evolved from magazines and VHS to a digitally delivered and inescapable behemoth, porn-star styling of the vulva conditioned boyfriends to pressure their girlfriends to mimic what they saw in porn. And the media hyped it up. Many of us wanted to be sexually 'wild' like a porn star. A whole culture grew around it – at Yumi's work, it became a thing to have a boozy lunch then go for a waxing.

Dr McCann agrees that pornography has had a huge influence, evolving from early 70s porn where a full bush was seen as a sign of sexiness, to what was literally described by *Hustler* magazine in 1975 as 'The Adolescent Look'. It marked the start of a change toward men seeing hairlessness as both desirable and associated with youthfulness. Dr McCann says, 'As a queer woman? I have literally never even seen a completely hairless vulva.'

Christina Zheng has no doubt that porn has created an expectation that women are groomed around the pubic area. 'I did have a weird, awkward experience. I was on a date and we went back to his place and we saw each other naked, and I could see that he felt a bit uncomfortable with me having a full bush. It was just a weird moment. Rightly or wrongly, I've carried that. I've wanted to eliminate that weirdness and that reaction from ever happening again.

'Sex with a new partner is awkward enough as it is. I want to remove any potential points of friction!'

As we know, the presence of pubic hair actually creates *less* friction in sex. But there are plenty of people who reckon sex is just better without pubes.

'I have a better sexual experience without pubes getting in the way,' says Christina. 'I feel sexier and am more easily stimulated. I'll do anything to give my partner a clear run at the target. Pubes also make oral sex a no-go zone. I'm not aroused by the idea of my husband sticking his face in a mountain of fur and getting pubes in his mouth. I want him to feel like he's going down in a fresh sourdough, not like he's frenching Chewbacca.'

Dr Uppal is all for women making choices about their bodies, but she does wish we'd all 'chill' a bit about our pubic hair. 'You don't need to remove it because it is cleaner, but if you feel better after removing it, then that's your personal choice. If that gives you joy or makes you feel more comfortable and that's the end product that you want for your body, then so be it.'

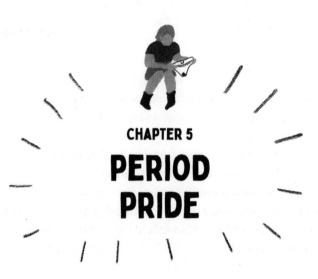

CHAPTER 5

PERIOD PRIDE

No matter your age or background, disgust and shame around periods never truly goes away. But is that aversion learnt – or is it 'natural'? And is it possible that even *you*, dear reader, are one of those people who are fearful and grossed out by your own period?

Alicia is 41 and the burn of shame from events that happened nearly 30 years ago still stings.

> When I was in Year 8 my male science teacher made fun of me in front of the whole class because we had cream dresses and I had leaked and didn't realise. The whole class laughed and he egged them on. I went to the office to get a spare dress and had tied my jumper around my waist (which was not allowed) so every teacher, male and female, that I passed stopped me to say, 'Take that jumper off!' and I had to explain why I couldn't and actually show them. What a dick teacher! – **ALICIA**

Sloane is 47, fabulous, open-minded and hilarious ... but still assuming there's an inherent turn-off in her 'bloody smell'.

> It was a frisky moment, and I had just gone down on him, so MY TURN! He didn't want to. I was at the end of my flow so I knew I wasn't gushing blood, but he didn't. I should've explained that to him, but then I thought, what if it smells a bit bloody down there and he's turned off forever? So I just ... moved on to penetration. I 100% need clitoral stimulation to orgasm so it took a lot of grinding on him to get me there, so he ended up with more blood in his pubes! But then I furiously wiped him off with 'the period sex' towel before he could sit up and see the brownish viscous love juice I'd deposited on his pubis. LOL. Too much information? – **SLOANE**

You might think that this aversion is to blood, not periods. But are you sure about that?

Imagine you're slicing vegetables for dinner. The knife slips and you cut your finger, but you're careful not to get blood in the food you are preparing.

Do you feel panic that your housemates might see your bleeding finger? Would you rush to the bathroom, embarrassed that your partner or kids saw blood on the counter? Do you treat the blood like a toxic contaminant, something that must be disposed of, hidden and disinfected? Do others in the house ignore you, knowing that you wouldn't want anyone to acknowledge you had just exposed a bloody finger? And, when you finally emerge having cleaned and covered your wound, do you pretend that it never happened?

Yeah ... it's just blood. Right?

Now let's take a moment to remember a time when your period leaked through your clothes. Maybe it was on your school uniform, like Alicia? Your work skirt? Your yoga pants? Did you get it on your boyfriend's sheets? Or worry that you left a smear behind on the rower at the gym?

Hold that thought for a minute and notice how your body is feeling. Do you feel ... crook? Is your heart racing a little, breath catching, stomach turning? That stress reaction means you can still feel a residue of shame in your body.

Sure, you may have an aversion to seeing blood, but our collective disgust for menstrual blood is something else altogether.

Ladies, we need to talk about our PERIODS.

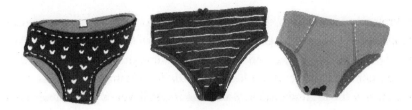

Your menstrual cycle is an incredible and complex series of bodily processes controlled by your brain, ovaries and several different hormones. It happens roughly once every month or so when your body prepares for pregnancy and the uterus lining (or endometrium) thickens. If there is no pregnancy, the endometrium starts to break down and come away from the uterus, which then triggers a period and resets the cycle. (Turn to page 90 for a 101 guide to your cycle.)

Like so much about your body, your cycle is unique. We have been told the norm is to get a period once every 28 days, but there is no standard length of a menstrual cycle. Claudine's cycle has been 21 to 25 days, while Yumi's sits fairly steadily at 28 days but can sometimes blow out to 35 and during one lockdown went on for a painful 57 days.

The average age for first a period (menarche) is 12–13 years, but again there is a fair degree of variation. Sometimes it can happen as young as 9 and other times it won't start until you're 16 or 17. As for menopause, the average age is about 51, but it can start anywhere from 40 (premature menopause) to later than 52 years (late menopause). Women's health organisation Jean Hailes estimates that **most women in Australia can expect to have between 450 and 500 periods.**

As an academic and researcher who focuses on the psychology of women's health, Professor Jane Ussher *loves* talking about periods. She loves them! She was desperate for her first period, which came when she was 12.

'I remember every month looking at my knickers and thinking, "When's it going to come?"'

We may be stating the bleeding obvious here, but when it comes to getting periods, enthusiasm and glee are *not* the typical reactions. It's usually the opposite.

'There's lots of different reasons for this,' says Professor Ussher. 'Some would say that it's to do with the abject female body – and everything in terms of the female body that's leaking and seeping and coming out of us as women – being seen as disgusting. So that would be menstruation, breastmilk, sweat ...'

Professor Ussher says this shame also comes from living in a culture of misogyny. 'It's positioning something that is essentially feminine as "other" and "dirty" and "disgusting" and a way of containing and controlling women.'

You don't have to look too hard to find a long history of periods being associated with dirt and disgust. Some cultures still worship the female body as the site of all creation, as was the case for some pre-religious societies, but there's not a lot of love for menstruation in most major religions, with menstruation often seen as impure, dirty or unhygienic. Some religions have strict rules and customs about what women can and can't do during their periods.

Jaime is 40, her parents are both Hindu Indian and she grew up in New Zealand. 'You couldn't go to any prayers or temple or religious events like Navratri if you had your period because you're considered dirty. You have to wait until it finishes, have a shower and wash your hair before you attend anything. Mum says it doesn't really happen anymore. It's kind of more historical because there was a real lack of education and now it's really different.

'I would go to my aunty's house, and she would get Grandma to come to the front door and ask me if I had my period because if I did she didn't want me to come in. She was quite religious. I can't remember being turned away, though. I probably lied and said I didn't have it! Because how would she know? And also I would've been embarrassed to say that I had my period.'

Dr Sneh Tiwari was born in Fiji, and she remembers periods were not talked about when she was a child. 'I'm the oldest child and the only girl in our family. Speaking about periods was and still is culturally taboo, especially in the presence of male relatives.'

Dr Tiwari knew nothing about periods right up until she had her first one. 'I was 13 years old and instead of explaining what it was, Mum placed emphasis on the practical management of the cycle like using the right underwear and homemade sanitary pads that had to be washed and hung to dry.'

Dr Tiwari is now a GP specialising in women's health, reproduction and mental health, but as a child no-one told her what was happening to her body and what it all meant. 'When there were only women together it was a slightly open discussion, and I remember when I was younger, my friends and I would use nicknames when talking about periods in the presence of other people.'

When you look at mainstream pop culture, periods are also pretty much ABSENT. Consider the hit 'reality' show *Survivor*, where castaway contestants are sent to an island with nothing but wilderness – and camera crews and sound recordists. In the 40 US seasons, the existence or management of periods was mentioned ONCE (Episode 1, Season 3, Africa).

It's astonishing that something we do, that you do, that 50 per cent of the world's population does, is considered so gross and shameful that our popular culture pretends *it just doesn't happen*! Like *that's* 'normal'!

You never see anyone on a screen looking for somewhere to throw their tampon, dry their period undies or wash out their cup, and you never see someone who has to quickly dash to the loo because their period has come early. Heaven forbid we see a bloodstained pair of undies! And that's just the tangible, visible stuff. What about the *Oh, I'm feeling moody because I'm about to get my period*? Or how about an office comedy where the main character gets a day off because her period pain is debilitating?

In her 20s, Claudine had atrocious period pain, and one night while working in a restaurant she had to lie down behind the coffee machine for 10 minutes in the middle of service. She remembers feeling utterly mortified that everyone would know she was bleeding, but the pain was so crippling she just couldn't stand up anymore.

Her normally quite shouty boss was so embarrassed he didn't know where to look and thought she was having a miscarriage. All the women she was working with knew exactly what was going on – and that she needed pain relief and a bed. In good news, her boss's awkwardness worked in her favour and he paid for her to take a cab home. But it was pretty uncomfortable the next day having to explain that she hadn't had a miscarriage, just period pain.

These moments are tediously common when you've got a uterus, and yet they leave us feeling defective, embarrassed and alone, feeling like, *Why can't I just manage this like everyone else?* The more difficult your periods, the more alone you feel and the harder it is to ask for help.

This collective effort to ignore the red elephant in the room means we're contributing to a culture of isolation and silence. It also makes it nigh on impossible to openly discuss the challenges our periods bring, except to our closest confidantes.

Why? 'Cos SHAME.

One thing Professor Ussher's research has shown is that young women from all kinds of backgrounds share a deep-rooted fear that someone will FIND OUT they are having their period.

And even worse than that? 'The worst thing is blood being *seen*.'

'This leads to menstrual shame that can be internalised by young women. This then has a really big impact not only on how they see their menstruating bodies, but also how they see their whole reproductive bodies. And this can have an impact on their sexuality.'

Even the most woke and accepting people in our feminist-podcast-loving community can be susceptible to shame.

Jess is a 37-year-old married lesbian who shared a story about an event that she described as 'mortifying'. 'I leaked last week ... at a party with people I didn't even know! I cried as it's not my first leaking and I always feel I already take too much space as a fat woman in this thin-loving world – to be a gross bleeder on furniture really hurt.'

Jess sent the hosts an apology message: *I've just been to the toilet and I'm mortified to see I'm a couple of days early ... I've made a big mess in the car and can only assume I have on your beautiful chairs as well ... please let me get them cleaned if I did. Or buy you a new chair. I'm absolutely mortified.*

'It was a Rainbow family dinner party so the hosts were two mums in their later years – one being a nurse – so they were really gracious and lovely.

'However, when I confided to my bestie she said, "Lucky you didn't do that at our place – Leon wouldn't be able to look you in the eye ever again." I know that wouldn't have been the case as Leon is practically family and would eventually laugh about it 'cos it's me and I'm "not normal" – but the fact that she said it made me feel even worse ... even though she thought she was joking!'

✳ ✳ ✳

Karen Pickering is a feminist writer and researcher who has surveyed thousands of girls and women for her book, *About Bloody Time,* co-written with political theorist Jane Bennett. One of the questions they asked was: 'What would make your experience of periods better?'

Many girls of school age responded with a pretty heartbreaking wish for pads and tampons with 'wrappers that don't make any sound'.

The survey reinforces anecdotal evidence that many young kids are getting limited information and education about their menstrual cycles, and what they are being taught focuses on HIDING any evidence that they are having a period.

Or, as Pickering says, they're learning to 'keep it a secret and [not] let anyone know they're struggling'.

This is why she wants to get evidence-based, non-commercial menstrual education into schools.

'A lot of mainstream education that's delivered, even in public schools, is by corporations. So companies that sell tampons and pads are the mode or the method by which young people are learning about menstruation. I think that has a lot of really big ethical problems.'

The way Yumi's mum taught her about periods was to hand her a brochure from a pad company. That was the entire chat.

In research involving women from a range of cultural backgrounds who migrated to Australia and Canada as refugees in the last decade, Professor Ussher and her colleagues found that many knew nothing about periods and were completely unprepared. They thought they were dying or something was really wrong with them.

'A really high percentage of women told us they didn't know about menstruation before their first period, so they felt horror, they felt shocked,' says Professor Ussher.

'As kids they didn't then go to their mother and say, "I'm dying!" They didn't tell anybody! They kept it secret. There was still a sense there was something wrong with them but also, "I'm not going to do anything about this, I'm not going to get help." A lot of it was experienced privately, with young women saying, "When I was a girl, I couldn't look at anybody. I went off in a room on my own. I cried."'

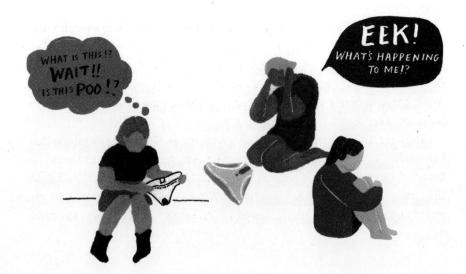

This is exactly what happened to Karalyn, a white woman who says, 'I had a mum and SIX AUNTIES and not one of them talked to me about puberty. When I got my period I had no idea what it was because my mum had not told me.'

Karalyn, by the way, is not from the olden days. She is 47 years old.

'I thought I had a disease. I thought I was sick. The blood wasn't red at first – it was that brown pasty discharge, so I thought it was poop! Then when the blood came in I thought the poop had hurt my vagina. I actually thought I might be dying. After about three days of terror I finally showed my mum my undies. She laughed – in that shameful/nervous way – gave me a pad, then rang all my aunties and her friends to tell them. I could hear her laughing with them.'

Professor Ussher says menstrual shame can be the starting point of a bigger cycle of shame, silence and secrecy that goes on to permeate our entire sexual and reproductive lives.

'Lack of knowledge about sex isn't uncommon,' says Professor Ussher. 'I have heard many women saying they didn't know about sex before they got married, and they didn't know what sex involved. So, they experience being horrified on their wedding night, being in a lot of pain, having no notion of their own sexual desire or pleasure, not having any notion of sexual rights, and very little knowledge around contraception, STIs and sexual health.

'I'm not saying menstrual shame is the cause of all of this, but it's a really significant part of a jigsaw.'

This shame can be passed on to the next generation when women have their own daughters. While they don't want to put their children through the same experience, they don't know how to talk to them about this thing that is culturally taboo.

Jenish is Nepalese from the Newar community. 'When I was a kid, if I had my period I was not allowed to sit at the dining table with the others. I had to sit on the floor and have my meal served to me. Finish it down there. And then I couldn't put my dishes with the rest – I had to wash my own dishes. And if there were any festivities or religious ceremonies, I was not allowed to participate for the four days of my period.

'Because that was the norm in the house, my aunties would do the same, my mother would do the same, so I didn't know the difference. As I grew up I started to understand. When my uncles married, two other aunties joined the family and they started to question, "Why do we have to do that?" But my grandparents were strict and enforced the rules. "If we don't follow the rules something bad might happen to the family! If we don't follow those rituals, somebody might fall ill or have an accident!"

'After my graduation ... my mum started feeling a bit more liberal and she would whisper, "Don't tell your grandma you have your period, just sit with us." She doesn't allow us to go to the temple, but she allows us to do whatever we want in the kitchen.'

Pickering agrees that the bigger-picture impact of secrecy, ignorance and the refusal to educate can be pretty devastating.

'The shame that girls and women are encouraged to feel around getting their period has massive knock-on effects for everyone in society. It affects women's body image. It can lead to things like self-harm and eating disorders. It can affect their sexual decision-making and their understanding of consent.'

A girl with an intellectual disability dropped a used pad from her underwear in science class in Year 8. She was teased about it relentlessly for months. She also used to leak blood on her school dress. After that a couple of us took her to Priceline to teach her what tampons were ... she had no idea how they worked. I don't think she ever got her period on her dress again after that. – **CASS**

Menstrual stigma and shame hits hardest for one particular group: those who live with period poverty.

Period poverty affects your ability to work, go to school and participate in social and cultural events. Around the world, millions of girls and women experience period poverty every month. It affects women in Australia too, in particular Indigenous girls and women living in remote communities and those in our communities who are already most vulnerable.

PERIOD POVERTY

Lack of access to menstrual products like pads and tampons (usually because they're unaffordable but also because they're unavailable), and lack of access to handwashing facilities, menstrual hygiene education and waste management.

Linda grew up in a conservative small town in WA. 'I never missed school or work but not being able to afford tampons affected my ability to play sport,' she says. 'I was very good at sport – a range of them – but sports uniforms were tight. I wasn't going to wear bloomers and a pad to basketball. I had to use a kitchen towel sometimes. And I stole tampons a few times. Usually from the school nurse, which I reasoned wasn't stealing.

'There were a few girls at my school who missed class because of period poverty. One girl often came to school without enough clothes and no lunch – she defo wasn't buying tampons. She "smelled" too, so I imagine periods made that worse.'

There is some good news though: there are moves to address period poverty and this is helping to open up the conversation around menstruation. In parts of Australia and around the world, schools are providing free menstrual products. Our hope is that by the time you read this book, all schools across Australia will have made free menstrual products available to those who need them.

In Tasmania, the state government decided to make pads and tampons available to all students after a Year 9 student from north Tasmania wrote to the education minister. Layla Seen knew some of her classmates weren't coming to school or were leaving early because they didn't have access to sanitary products at home.

In January 2021, Isobel Marshall was named Young Australian of the Year for her work to end period poverty and menstrual stigma. Marshall and her best friend Eloise Hall created a social enterprise that sells organic pads and tampons in Australia and sends the profits overseas to help provide women with access to sustainable sanitary healthcare and education.

During her acceptance speech, Marshall told a room full of politicians and leaders – many of them older men in suits – that 'periods should not be a barrier to education. They should not cause shame, and menstrual products should be accessible and affordable. They are not a luxury or a choice.'

Later during the awards ceremony, hip-hop artist Nardean performed a poem (called 'Miracles' – you can find it on YouTube) that painted a word picture of period shame and the stigma around bleeding. She ended her poem with the line, 'Today I am proud to walk with rubies in between my legs.'

When the cameras panned the crowd, there were a few people fidgeting in their seats (mostly older men in suits), but there were many more women quietly nodding their heads with a deep sense of recognition.

✳ ✳ ✳

'It was the most badass and most comfortable choice for my own body.'

Remember back in 2015 when images of Kiran Gandhi running the London Marathon – with the patch of period blood between her legs visibly growing bigger through her leggings with each mile she ran – went viral and sparked international debate?

'I knew it would be a radical move,' says Kiran. 'I knew it was combating stigma and my own shame in my own right. But I didn't know how powerful it would be.'

Yumi had a strong reaction to the images. When she first saw stories about Kiran pop up in her newsfeed, she closed the lid on her laptop. But the algorithms did their job. It came up again. And again. And eventually, she looked. It was confronting. But there was something bold and wonderful in the photos of Kiran joyfully crossing the marathon's finish line, arms linked with two of her friends, with her blood unhidden and unashamed.

'I was like, "Damn! I'm running and bleeding!"' says Kiran. 'Women do extraordinary things all over the world and I felt an enormous sense of power. Any person bleeding from anywhere and running a marathon is a punk rock move that commands the respect of everyone, and women are doing far more extraordinary things than this daily. So it was like, "Man, we have so much love to give to the women in our lives instead of this misogyny forcing us to shroud this stuff in silence."'

This was the opposite of period shame. This was PERIOD PRIDE.

The reason Yumi didn't want to confront the photos of Kiran was because she'd never seen it before. She literally became a full-grown adult before she saw what it would look like for someone to ... *free bleed*. And you know what? It wasn't bad at all. It was just a bit of blood.

During the marathon, Kiran heard people muttering that she was bleeding, as though she hadn't noticed, and a woman tried to shame her for bleeding through her tights, but Kiran decided to pay no mind. 'The second that we accept our own shame, people are able to come and do that to us. The second you own it, no-one can really shame you. You put a protective bubble around yourself.'

Yumi went on to co-write a guidebook to getting your period with Dr Melissa Kang called *Welcome to Your Period*. The whole point of the book is to normalise menstruation, arm young kids with the info they need, and tell the truth about periods. That, yeah, everyone has a spill and a leak – and you absolutely won't die of shame when it happens. The book probably wouldn't have happened if Yumi hadn't interviewed Kiran for *Ladies, We Need To Talk*.

And the feedback Yumi gets on that book? Every woman who gets it for her daughter says the same thing: 'I wish I'd had this book when I was a kid.'

Partly because of the huge reaction to her run, and partly because she is a radical feminist, Kiran Gandhi has given a lot of thought to period stigma. 'Women have long been valued for our looks, as opposed to our skill sets. And so when you have something like a period, which is not sexually consumable or enjoyable, in the same way our beauty is, or our breasts or our personalities, are ... we're made to be ashamed of it and hide it away, like it doesn't exist. And that's completely oppressive.'

It makes you wonder: how can we all flip that shame? And what would it be like to live without it?

No more worrying about the noise your tampon wrapper makes. Swimming on a hot day, even if it's the first day of your period. Saying, 'Hey, I'm bleeding but I still want to have sex.' Leaving your box of pads on the counter instead of hiding them in the back of a drawer. Washing your menstrual cup in the bathroom sink in front of someone. Or saying, 'I can't – I'm bleeding too heavily today.'

Professor Ussher cites the work of Karen Horney, who was a feminist psychoanalyst whose theories questioned traditional Freudian views. 'Her argument was that a lot of the negative cultural discourses around menstruation are actually born from misogyny, which is actually based on fear of women.

'Because to have the power to reproduce is such an incredible power. To have a womb, to be able to give birth. If we take a step back from it, it's not an illness. Menstruation is not a curse. It's actually a sign of incredible power.'

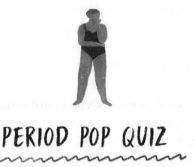

PERIOD POP QUIZ

1. You can't fall pregnant if you have sex during your period.

   A. True

   B. False

2. Which of the following hormones is not involved in menstruation?

   A. Progesterone

   B. Adrenaline

   C. Follicle stimulating hormone (FSH)

   D. Oestrogen

3. What is menstrual blood made up of?

   A. It's the same as regular blood

   B. A mixture of blood, cervical mucus, vaginal secretions and endometrial tissue

   C. It doesn't contain any blood

   D. Lining cells of the vagina

4. On average, how much fluid does a woman release during her period?

   A. About two tablespoons, or 40 millilitres

   B. About five tablespoons, or 100 millilitres

   C. About a cup, or 250 millilitres

   D. About half a litre

5. **What is the most common cause of period pain?**
  - **A.** The release of an egg from the ovary
  - **B.** The contraction of muscles in the uterus
  - **C.** A build-up of menstrual fluid in the uterus
  - **D.** A woman's imagination

6. **When should you speak to your doctor about your periods?**
  - **A.** If there are changes in your cycle, such as bleeding more than normal or at unusual times
  - **B.** If you have regular pain in your pelvis that is not related to your period, or if you have pain during sex, or pain related to going to the toilet (either wee or poo)
  - **C.** If you have period pain that doesn't ease when you take ibuprofen or the pill (so if it's enough to stop you from going to work or school)
  - **D.** If you have symptoms that interfere with your ability to do normal things like go to school or work
  - **E.** If you are getting severe period pain that you have never had before, or period pain that gets significantly worse, after the age of 18
  - **F.** If you have pain or other symptoms, or if you have a mum or sister who has endometriosis
  - **G.** All of the above

ANSWERS

1. **B.** It doesn't happen often, but it can happen. Women can ovulate during or soon after they get their period, and sperm can live for several days once they are inside a woman. So your period isn't a free pass to forget contraception (and your period does nothing to protect you from STIs).

2. **B.** The main hormones involved in menstruation are oestrogen and progesterone (produced by the ovaries), and follicle stimulating hormone (FSH) and luteinising hormone (LH) (released by the pituitary gland in the brain).

3. **B.** We often think of menstrual fluid as just regular blood, but it's actually a mixture of tissues and secretions from inside the uterus, including blood, endometrial tissue, cervical mucus and vaginal secretions.

4. A. While the bleeding in a period can last several days to a week, on average you only lose about 40 millilitres (or two tablespoons) of period fluid. But anything between 5 millilitres (one teaspoon) and 80 millilitres (a third of a cup) is considered normal. Any more than 80 millilitres is considered excessive.

The best way to gauge the amount of fluid you are losing is to note the number of tampons or pads you use per day. If you are using more than 10 tampons or pads in a day (or you have to change a super pad or tampon more than every two hours) then that is considered excessive bleeding and worth following up with your GP.

5. B. There are known physical causes of period pain, the most common being an increased sensitivity to hormone-like fatty acids called prostaglandins, which are produced around menstruation. Prostaglandins cause contractions of the uterine muscles and other internal muscles, such as the bowel, stomach and blood vessels.

These contractions are what you feel during period pain, and yes, they're similar to the contractions that push a baby out during labour. During menstruation they help to cut off blood supply to the endometrium, reduce blood loss and push the menstrual fluid out of the vagina. Because that 'push' effect also works on the bowel, it can result in more poo than usual. The increased prostaglandins can lead to constipation and diarrhoea, nausea and vomiting, and pallor.

Sometimes there's an underlying condition causing pain that needs further investigation by a doctor, and treatment. You can also get pain mid-cycle when you ovulate (otherwise known as mittelschmerz), but this is different to period pain.

6. G. If you have any of these experiences, or ever just feel like something isn't right, it's worth talking to your doctor. (If you're feeling a bit uneasy talking to your doctor about your periods, we have some tips in chapter 12 on how to best prepare for and have those conversations.)

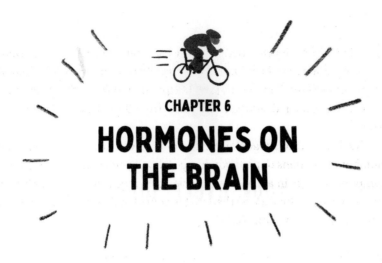

CHAPTER 6

HORMONES ON THE BRAIN

s it that time of the month? Are you on the rag? Are you getting your period or something? Are there any more dismissive and infuriating questions? They make us want to flip tables, or the finger, at the idiot who asked.

We don't usually get this easily irritated but we're feeling quite ... *testy* at the moment.

People assuming that hormones, PMS or your period are at play when you're feeling fed up, pissed off or fierce – what a bunch of class-A bullshit! It implies you have no control of your emotions, or yourself.

There's also an uncomfortable truth in these moments, because many of us are familiar with that sense of being possessed by a bad-tempered, gloomy and monstrous version of ourselves. You feel rage. You feel despair. You feel your family or colleagues are exasperating. And your desire for hot chips is insatiable.

And it feels very real ... because *it is* real.

But what often happens is, a day or two of feeling these feelings goes by, and then – like it's never happened before and we're taken by surprise – we bleed into our underpants, realise we've got our period, and within hours the grumpy mood has dissipated.

Awww, I was just premenstrual!

The hormones that form part of our cycle can affect our moods, social skills, productivity, horniness, our experience of pain ... among many other things.

Ladies, we need to talk about our HORMONES.

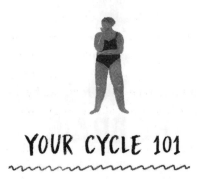

YOUR CYCLE 101

Your menstrual cycle is a very complex system that involves your brain, various organs and glands, and a bunch of hormones that travel via your bloodstream to relevant glands and organs. As we mentioned in the previous chapter, each menstrual cycle is unique, but most last between 21 and 35 days (28 days is considered average), and they are marked by four distinct phases.

1. **Menstruation** or DAY ONE of your period marks the beginning of your cycle. Your period usually lasts anywhere from three days to a week. It is the 'clean up' after your previous cycle, when you shed the lining of your uterus through your vagina.

2. **Follicular phase** begins on the first day of menstruation and ends with ovulation; it includes the days of your period and the week or so that follows. This stage is kicked off when a part of your brain (the hypothalamus) releases a follicular stimulating hormone (FSH). This hormone stimulates one of your ovaries to produce a number of follicles (from 5 to 20) that will sit on the surface of the ovary. Each follicle contains an immature egg (or ovum), but in most cases only one of these follicles matures into an egg. The growth of these follicles stimulates the lining of the uterus (the endometrium), which thickens to prepare for a pregnancy. This follicular phase is marked by a rise in the levels of oestrogen, which then prompts the release of other reproductive hormones that leads to ovulation.

3. **Ovulation** usually occurs smack-bang in the middle of the cycle, approximately two weeks before the beginning of the next period. It is less of a 'phase' and more of a 'moment', lasting around 12–24 hours, and involves the release of the mature egg from the surface of the ovary and into the fallopian tubes towards the uterus. This egg usually survives for about 24 hours and dies unless it is fertilised by a sperm. The follicle remains on the surface of the ovary, after the egg bursts from it.

4. **Luteal phase** lasts for about two weeks after ovulation. Once the egg has left the surface of the ovary, the follicle transforms and becomes the corpus luteum, which starts releasing progesterone and small amounts of oestrogen in order to help the uterus to create a thick lining in which a fertilised egg implants. If there isn't a pregnancy then the corpus luteum starts to break down around three-quarters of the way through the cycle, and progesterone levels drop.

THE MENSTRUAL CYCLE
(USING 28 DAYS AS AN EXAMPLE)

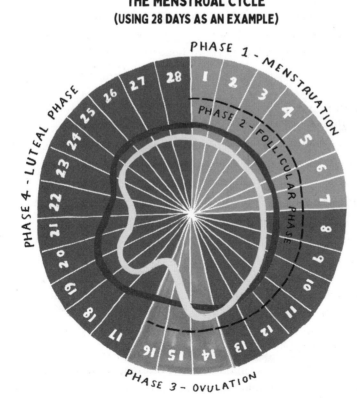

There are a bunch of hormones involved in your menstrual cycle, but when we talk about 'your hormones' we tend to be referring to the main reproductive hormones: oestrogen and progesterone. These are the ones that can have the most profound effect on your mental health.

Oestrogen is responsible for stimulating the growth of the lining of the uterus and it triggers the release of other hormones that kick off ovulation. As far as your mental health goes (and this is simplifying drastically), oestrogen is considered a 'good hormone'. Times in your cycle when oestrogen levels are high and stable tend to coincide with positive moods, and better concentration and memory. On average, you get two oestrogen peaks during your cycle.

Progesterone is a hormone that some of us have a more complicated relationship with, and it tends to be linked to depression and low mood. Part of this is about the 'dose' or amount of progesterone at different points in your cycle, but it's also about the fluctuations at different times and how individual women's brain chemistry interacts with the progesterone levels. Progesterone peaks in the second half of a cycle. But, because this is a very complex system, higher and more stable levels of progesterone can mean you are less anxious.

Not all of us are sensitive to these hormones and their fluctuations across our cycles, so your experience of the physical, mental and emotional impact of hormonal changes will be different to others.

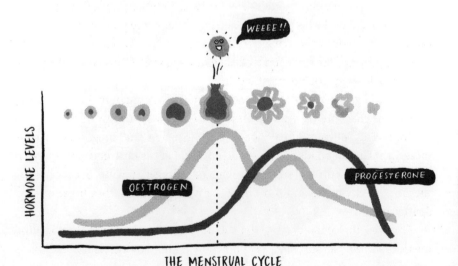

THE MENSTRUAL CYCLE

Let's think about the hormones in our cycle using ... cycles. Imagine that the hormones oestrogen and progesterone are chemical bicycle messengers carrying information around your body. They carry messages from your brain to your uterus, ovaries and the rest of your body, and back again. At different times in your cycle, there's a variation in the level of your hormones – or, in other words, the number of bike messengers whizzing around changes.

At the beginning of your cycle, when you're menstruating, you're going to struggle to find any bike messengers. There's only a few, and an equal amount of oestrogen and progesterone messengers. The roads are mostly calm and you feel fairly relaxed.

Dr Rosie Worsley – not a bike messenger, but an endocrinologist whose work focuses on women's hormones and health – says that most of us feel pretty good after the first day or so of our period. But we all respond differently to fluctuations in hormones so it's not a hard-and-fast rule. (You will probably notice this change more if you've had a really rough lead-up to your period.)

As you continue further into the follicular phase, your oestrogen levels increase. This means there are more oestrogen bike messengers on the road, while most of the progesterone messengers are still locked in the bike shed.

The oestrogen messengers are fast, efficient and polite on the roads. They can help you feel good about yourself and get heaps done. And as you get closer to ovulation, you may notice that some of the messages the bike folks are sending are making you feel ... kinda hot and horny.

Next comes ovulation, which is the moment the ripest egg is released from one of your ovaries. This moment is a distinct marker at the halfway point of your menstrual cycle. It's physically detectable for some people by an ache in one of their ovaries or a change in vaginal discharge – when the mucus gets most slippery and stretchy and looks like raw egg white. This is also the point in your cycle when you are most fertile.

Then things get quieter for a bit. Some of the oestrogen messengers head back to the shed, but on the whole the vibe is still fairly positive.

That is until your luteal phase. This is when the progesterone bike messengers hit the roads en masse and outnumber the oestrogen messengers. How you react to progesterone messengers depends on you. For some of us, they're perfectly polite and stay out of our way. For others, they bring misery, apathy and rage.

Amid all this chaos, a big (red) alarm sounds. The progesterone bike messengers, whose numbers have been dwindling anyway, leave, and we're left with the turmoil.

Before we go any further, let's be clear on what we mean when we talk about PMS or premenstrual syndrome.

PMS involves a mix of physical, mental and emotional symptoms that some of us experience in the lead up to menstruation – so when the progesterone bike messengers are all out on the roads.

For them to 'count' as PMS, these symptoms usually end just before or soon after you get your period, and you have at least one week symptom free before they start up again midway through your cycle. If they don't follow this pattern, your symptoms are likely being caused by something else.

The list of PMS symptoms is long (some sources say there are up to 150) so we won't list them all, but the most common are:

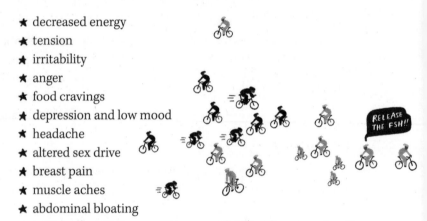

* decreased energy
* tension
* irritability
* anger
* food cravings
* depression and low mood
* headache
* altered sex drive
* breast pain
* muscle aches
* abdominal bloating
* oedema (swelling caused by excess fluid) of fingers and ankles

RELEASE THE FSH!!

Most figures suggest about 80 per cent of us get PMS. The majority of us will only get a small selection of PMS symptoms, which are not fun and a bit disruptive, but we can still go about our lives.

A few days out from her period, Claudine starts obsessing about cake and crunchy baguettes (food cravings), keeps losing her keys and glasses (difficulty focusing) and gets grumpy at her family (irritability). Yumi has a couple of days where she utterly loathes her partner (anger and irritability) and feels despondent about her life choices (depression and low mood). Then we bleed and things return to normal with few consequences. We know heaps of other women who have similar experiences.

But for a small group of women, crushing hormone-related mood changes can make life completely bloody miserable.

DEALING WITH PMS

Like period pain, PMS symptoms don't have to be stoically endured. There's a lot that can be done to alleviate how awful you feel. Not everything works for everyone, so expect to try a few things out in different combos to see what works for you.

Track your cycle with a calendar, diary or app. Seeing the alert on your phone or the marking on the page can help you feel a little seen, snap out of your funk or at least acknowledge that, *Yes, it's true that I detest everything right now, but it's also true that right now I have PMS.*

Exercise! Exercising gives you access to possibly THE greatest party drug of all time: endorphins. Having tried quite a few, Yumi recommends this drug. If you get a good hit of endorphins, you can recover from the grumps, feel accomplished, and reduce fatigue and depression. Exercise and eating (read on) can also help manage period pain.

Eat some foods, avoid others. All the usual stuff. Eat more calcium, leafy greens, whole grains, fruit and veg. Avoid caffeine, salty food, highly processed foods, anything that might add to your bloat (and if bloating is a major problem, think about eating smaller portions of food more often). Chamomile, raspberry leaf or other herbal teas might also have a soothing effect.

Talk to a counsellor. Cognitive Behavioural Therapy, a counselling technique used for treating depression, can help women better understand how hormonal changes throughout the menstrual cycle affect their thinking and mood and provide them with strategies for coping.

Talk to your GP on whether you might benefit from a supplement. While there isn't a lot evidence supporting their use, some women find supplements helpful. Vitex agnus-castus (or chaste tree), vitamin B6, evening primrose oil and calcium supplements may ease some PMS symptoms. Doctors may also recommend you use other medication, including adjusting birth control.

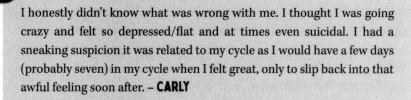

> From the moment I ovulate to when I start bleeding, I see the world through a darker lens. I feel bleak and despairing, have trouble coping with daily life and cry a lot. For the other 10 days, I'm solid and stable and optimistic, and often start projects or initiate activities that I later dread. I'm seeing someone new, and for part of the month I feel like calling it off, and for the other part I'm all for it. It's a really tiring struggle, and it's been going on for decades, although I've only recently mapped it against my cycle. I wonder how many women out there go through the same thing? – **BRYONY**

What Bryony described has the hallmarks of a condition known as premenstrual dysphoric disorder (PMDD). According to Jean Hailes, PMDD affects 3 to 8 per cent of people who menstruate. Symptoms include extreme difficulty concentrating, depression, anxiety and panic attacks, tiredness and marked lack of energy, sleep issues, feeling overwhelmed, and increased thoughts of suicide and self-harm.

Bryony's email was the first of many we've received. The emails all had similar stories of being absolutely hammered by mental health issues in the second part of a menstrual cycle. And they *all* include stories of women who struggled to get their healthcare professionals to take them seriously.

> I honestly didn't know what was wrong with me. I thought I was going crazy and felt so depressed/flat and at times even suicidal. I had a sneaking suspicion it was related to my cycle as I would have a few days (probably seven) in my cycle when I felt great, only to slip back into that awful feeling soon after. – **CARLY**

Professor Jayashri Kulkarni is a psychiatrist and researcher who's spent decades working in women's mental health. She is pushing for a better understanding of how our reproductive hormones can affect our mental health.

'The same hormones – oestrogen and progesterone – that are in charge of ovulation and having babies are also in charge of whether you're depressed, anxious, angry or have foggy brain,' says Professor Kulkarni.

'What we talk about, particularly with perimenopausal depression, PMDD, or even PMS, is brain sensitivity. Everyone has hormone fluctuations. But some hormone fluctuations really react on the brain chemistry and the brain circuitry in some women.

'For these women even tiny fluctuations can cause a real dip in mood. Whereas other women can have the same or bigger fluctuations and not have any mental health effect.'

Professor Kulkarni talks about a 'spectrum' of mental health issues that can be caused by fluctuations in our reproductive hormones across our menstrual cycles. 'I see PMS at the lesser end and PMDD at the severe end. There are similarities – PMS usually presents with more physical symptoms. Bloating, breast swelling, tenderness, a bit of sadness, a bit of brain fog, but not much. Just sort of generally feeling yucky and irritable.

'But PMDD looks different. That pattern of sudden onset of change in thinking, change in behaviour, change in mood, and sudden offset as well.'

Professor Kulkarni can spot PMDD a mile off. In her clinic she sees women who are quite unwell and know something is not right. They often turn up to their first appointment with their own documentation – notes on their phones, folders of records, journals of menstrual cycles and interviews with female family members. For many of her patients, learning that their hormones may be the cause of their suffering can be a huge relief.

'Even knowing that this is going on, and it's got a biological basis to it, is sometimes really comforting for people to understand.'

On average it takes 12 years to get a diagnosis of PMDD, according to the 2018 Global Survey of PMDs (Premenstrual Disorders). Many women experience years of having their symptoms dismissed or written off as 'normal PMS', not only by their colleagues, friends and families, but also by health professionals.

'It's really awful that so many women have been told they're inadequate, they're pathetic, it's all in their heads, or it's an excuse for bad behaviour,' says Professor Kulkarni.

This is not unusual for women's health conditions or mental illness in general, but what makes PMDD particularly challenging to diagnose is that there's NO SINGLE STORY about how our hormones affect our mental health. There's no consistent experience. We all have unique brain chemistry.

In the podcast, we spoke to Fiona, whose PMDD began after the birth of her first child. 'From days 14 to 28 I felt like I was a different person. I was non-functional, a lot of days couldn't get out of bed. Or when I did, I was really manic, very hyper. Huge amounts of energy, but huge amounts of rage as well. Just a nightmare to be around for friends and family, unfortunately.'

Fiona was diagnosed with polycystic ovarian syndrome as well as postnatal depression, but the treatments she was given didn't work and she was still unwell. She describes feeling like a guinea pig, having tests and treatments that she knew were unlikely to help her.

'I would do all the treatments required to treat those illnesses and I would still have issues. We did a lot of blood tests and hormone profiling, and it showed that I was very deficient in progesterone. So they would supplement me with progesterone and that made things 10 times worse.'

In an experience that matches what Professor Kulkarni has seen, Fiona struggled to get the right diagnosis and treatment.

'That was probably the most disheartening and frustrating part of the whole ordeal – trying to have someone that actually believed in it. This was only five years ago, and there just really weren't that many people who had heard about [PMDD]. They thought it was purely a mental health disorder. So they would say, "Go see a counsellor, go see a psychologist, go on antidepressants, diet, exercise," all of those things. I had covered off a lot of those bases from any sort of holistic approach I could. To no effect.

'It was really, really hard to actually get someone that was willing to help me. *Really* help me.'

Some of us have brain chemistry that makes us more sensitive to hormonal changes. So those times in our lives when our hormone levels are *fluctuating* can make some of us more vulnerable to PMS, PMDD and to mood disorders, including anxiety. At certain times in our reproductive lives – including pregnancy and the postnatal period, perimenopause and menopause – changes in hormone levels can really affect mood.

While Professor Kulkarni has seen girls as young as 10, many of the women she sees only start to experience PMDD symptoms in their 30s or 40s.

'I've heard this so many times. "I was OK. I used to have a bit of period pain, it was just a bit niggly, a little bit of a headache here and there, but not that much. And now, after my second baby, every cycle, I have this crash." I've heard that so many times that I don't think it's just coincidence.'

No-one knows for sure what causes PMDD, but genetics, environment and relationships are believed to play a role. Professor Kulkarni thinks that for some women hormonal changes during pregnancy may play a role.

'Because it is a dynamic system, it gets set at different levels like a thermostat. So perhaps with the pregnancies there's a whole bundle of changes, and it never quite goes back to exactly the same setting in terms of the sensitivity of the brain chemistry to the hormonal shifts.'

Sometimes a woman's diagnosis will trigger a family conversation, at which point it emerges that generations of female family members have had similar experiences. But they never felt they could talk about it.

Professor Kulkarni also suspects other experiences may play a role. 'What I keep seeing in my clinic is that women who have had early life trauma or abuse tend to be the ones who experience worse PMDD. They seem to be more sensitive to perinatal or postnatal depression and have a worse experience of menopause.'

Her theory is that early trauma triggers the release of stress hormones, including cortisol, and this affects the developing brain's biochemistry, making the person more sensitive to reproductive hormones.

'It might be that I'm seeing a select group, because I'm seeing people as a second-opinion psychiatry clinic and people come because they have mental health issues. And mental health issues themselves are often rooted in stuff that happened back then.'

But what is clear is that a diagnosis can be a turning point for many women with PMDD.

'It's not made up. It's not a woman behaving badly. It's important to educate the other people in the woman's life: partners, parents, family and whoever else. Everyone needs to stop stigmatising this person by saying it's all in her head and she's just making it up.'

Not only does a diagnosis help a woman, and those in her life, to better understand what is going on; it can also mean getting closer to the right treatment. One of the aims of treatment is to stabilise hormones so that the brain isn't exposed to those different doses throughout the cycle – or, returning to our earlier analogy, to keep a fairly consistent number of bike messengers on the road at all times.

Dr Worsley says certain contraceptive pills can work well for some women, but it has to be the right pill for the individual. The *wrong* pill could make things worse! She also uses low-dose antidepressants on some patients and finds that they too can really help.

'In PMDD some women are actually able to use the antidepressants only for two weeks out of the month rather than all the time. They seem to respond much quicker to it as opposed to in depression. Classically, in depression, you're told, "Well, it might take four to six weeks to work." In one PMDD study, symptoms like irritability started improving within about 14 hours.'

While it's not entirely clear why this is the case, Dr Worsley says it could be that the antidepressants are helping the brain respond better to the hormone fluctuations.

When we released our episode on 'The Secret Life of Hormones', Carly wrote to us to say her GP sent her to an endocrinologist who prescribed low-dose antidepressants, which helped her 'feel like myself again!'

Fiona decided that she needed to take a different, more drastic course of action. 'I had a radical hysterectomy. So I had my uterus, my cervix, my ovaries, everything removed.'

While Fiona admits it was an extreme decision to make at 35, it's one she absolutely stands by. 'I was fortunate enough to have one child. I had a very difficult pregnancy and I knew I wouldn't be able to carry again. They actually put me into surgical menopause for six months, where they implant a little blocker inside your tummy. I had that for six months to prove that the illness was in fact cycle-related and hormone-related. I was great during that time.'

There were a number of other hoops she had to jump through in order to have the surgery, but she believes that advocating for herself and going ahead with it saved her life. 'Now I have my life back for the first time in six, seven years. I'm a very happy single parent and it's amazing. I'm very, very, very fortunate.'

Alex* was on the pill from when she was a teenager, and then decided to take a break from it. 'Over the course of maybe five years I realised I was super anxious and depressed for one to two weeks of my cycle after I ovulated. I tried everything – excessive exercise, cutting out sugar, two different contraceptive pills, period tracking apps and acupuncture – but I always felt out of control during this period. I really wanted to deal with things "naturally" but it kept getting the better of me.

'After the episode on "The Secret Life of Hormones", I thought *fuck it* and spent the $360 and finally saw an endocrinologist/gynaecologist. He prescribed a couple of different contraceptive pills, all of which I tried and had annoying reactions to. The next thing he suggested was a vaginal ring and it has changed my life. I've been using it for about six months and I feel 100 per cent more level and in control of my life.'

✳ ✳ ✳

There is an uncomfortable tension around this biological perspective of women's mental health. That's because of the long-held – and SEXIST – view that our hormones make us inherently irrational, emotional and unable to control our behaviour and thinking. This argument is often used to suggest that women are biologically unsuited for certain jobs, activities, and even rights.

This is something Professor Kulkarni feels conflicted about. Growing up, she too heard the 'classic sexist crap' like 'you can't talk to her because she's on her rags'. But after her decades of clinical work and research, Professor Kulkarni believes it is clear that helping women to better understand their bodies, including their hormones, empowers them.

'What we're saying is, understand why you feel like crap, because there is a solution. If you're feeling this terrible depression that's premenstrual, then you can seek help for that.

'Then you can tell everyone to shut up if they try and do pejorative stuff to you – but also say, "There's much more to me than my hormones, and once I get that under control, then there's no stopping me!"'

Professor Jane Ussher, psychologist of women's health with decades of research and clinical experience (we met her in the periods chapter), is an excellent person to bring into this conversation about hormones and the brain. She has a different view. 'I would say it's *not* purely a biological thing. There's much more going on.'

Professor Ussher doesn't deny that some women experience PMDD, but she's wary of the suggestion that hormones are a key driver of women's mental health challenges. Her research suggests our experience of premenstrual symptoms is very much influenced by the rest of our lives – our work, relationships, frustrations, the laundry piles.

When Professor Ussher interviewed women with PMS and asked whether their symptoms were different when they were away from their daily stressors and on holiday, the women often responded with, 'Actually ... it's not as bad.'

'There's almost a physiological vulnerability ... that can make us much more sensitive to what's happening around us,' says Professor Ussher. 'It's like a greater reactivity [to hormones]. But if you take those pressures off, then actually, you're not necessarily that reactive.'

Professor Ussher adds, 'So many women have said to me, "It's my real feelings that come out at that time. All that stuff I bottle up for three weeks of the month. All that being good, being nice, putting up with stuff. I feel fucking furious when I'm premenstrual and that's righteous anger that actually feels good."

'We found that women self-silence for three weeks of the month, and then when they're premenstrual it's like they either can't or won't self-silence anymore.'

It's an interesting point to consider. Claudine can experience some pretty nasty PMS, especially in the dark cold depths of winter, but she can't ever remember having it when she's been on holidays at her favourite beach (and she's definitely had periods there). When the house is messy and the kids are being annoying and her period is on its way, Yumi has a feeling of impending eruption, like a lifetime of suppressed fury wants to burst out in enormous geysers of menstrual fluid, red-hot and visible from outer space. But if she's alone in a peaceful, clean space? No PMS!

Anger, whether it's righteous or otherwise, is something women are not supposed to feel and so we put a lid on it. We bite our tongue when our colleague says something offensive, shrug it off when our partner asks why there isn't any milk in the fridge, and keep our cool every day when we come home and the lounge room is a mess of bags, dirty socks and lunch boxes. This all adds up, day in, day out. Oh yeah, and then there's systemic discrimination! We have a few things to be pissed off about.

Professor Ussher says we have the right to be angry and 'we shouldn't have to attribute it to our hormones'.

> 'If you're a woman who gets really angry, that's not allowed, because you're hysterical, you're menopausal or you're premenstrual, whereas when a man gets really angry, it's like, OK, there must be a legitimate reason for it.'

She has developed a psychological therapy that encourages women to think more deeply about their anger and not self-censor during the rest of their cycle. She's also developed a form of couples therapy that helps partners to understand the bigger picture of what's going on, at all times of the menstrual cycle.

One of the aims is to help all people learn that for those of us with a uterus, certain feelings and behaviours are likely to change across the cycle, and there are ways to help us understand what's going on at that moment that aren't dismissive or demeaning.

Understanding how you are affected by your cycle can help you plan your life to utilise the good and the bad and the in-between. We can make the most of it by working WITH what's happening to our bodies instead of struggling against it or pretending like it's not happening.

Professor Ussher's message is twofold: general improvements to life quality can reduce sensitivity to hormones; and just because mood swings are attached to your cycle, it doesn't mean they're not valid.

'The therapy helps the woman to express her feelings and needs throughout the whole cycle, and helps the woman to take time for herself, rather than just caring for everyone all the time.'

Do YOU need help expressing your feelings? Here are some clapbacks when annoying people ask if you're on your period.

Why? Are you a vampire?

No, I'm just like this when I'm around annoying people.

Please go away, you're wasting my will to live.

Yes, OMG, the blood clots are the size of a small apple. Do you want to see?

Don't talk to me unless you come bearing doughnuts. And hot chips.

Why are you talking to me?

Do you need a tampon? Hold on a sec, I'm pretty sure I have one in here.

Yes and I'll bleed on everything you love.

Why? Are you suffering from womb envy?

You thirsty?

Yes. And anything you can do, I can do bleeding.

No mate, my vagina is fine. Thanks for asking.

MAKE YOUR CYCLE WORK FOR YOU

One way to get a better sense of how your hormones affect you is to chart your cycle for a few months and figure out what is normal for you. It is difficult to apply if your periods are irregular but, as we've flagged, your menstrual cycle can be roughly broken up into four stages. If you imagine your cycle is exactly 28 days long, breaking it into four phases will give you one week per phase. We've mapped our cycles here as an example, along with Kim* and Lisa.

	YUMI	CLAUDINE
PHASE 1	After the heaviest bleeding day, apathy is quickly replaced by thinking big, planning ahead, feeling athletic, positive, sociable, plus a reduced appetite.	The first day or so of the period is a bit crampy and blah. Then things can feel more promising, but it does depend on what else is happening. 'Cos post-period hormones aren't enough to shift my mood if there are other things making me anxious.
PHASE 2	Making things happen, wanting sex, feeling creative, expansive and excited.	A bit of extra energy and enthusiasm here, but not as much as other women seem to experience.
PHASE 3	Still wanting sex, feeling horny, loving everyone, harmonious work relationships, merriment.	More interested in sex. More forgiving.
PHASE 4	Hating partner, feeling glum and worthless, eating awful snacks, avoiding people, feeling poorly and needing naps.	Feeling quite irritated and frustrated that NO-ONE puts their stuff away. More likely to get weepy about everything.

	LISA	**KIM**
VITAL INFO	Has always had debilitating periods.	Has pretty intense PMDD, which got worse as she got older, and her cycle never fit the standard four-phases pattern.
PHASE 1	Whole body aches for a day or so. Feel a bit whatever. Bleeding too heavy to do anything really. No appetite, just eat to replenish (my 'pho' phase 'cos I'll eat a pho). Sometimes the bleeding's so bad I leak onto the train seat or the chair at work. By day four I'm exhausted with the blood loss and take a few days to recuperate.	No two cycles are the same. Follicular, ovulation and luteal phase were all like luteal phase. Start to bleed and feel 'normal' for a few days, maybe two weeks. The few good days during menstruation were the only respite, when my ovaries were 'at rest'. Sometimes only one or two symptom-free days.
PHASE 2	Can do anything and am amazing and funny and really nice and supportive of everyone. Sex is great. Re-embrace keeping fit and exercising.	Then could have two weeks just feeling anaesthetised and bloated, which meant period was on its way. Some months could 'feel' the
PHASE 3	Sex is still good, everything fun and easy. Basically got a 'good attitude'. Wonder, was all that PMS stuff even real?	change as it occurred – dread, then tears, knowing the despair was coming back. Sometimes felt rage, and I'd rip someone's head off.
PHASE 4	Boobs get massive and sore (need to wear two bras). Nighttime anxiety creeps in. Also SO hungry. Like, pregnant hungry. Start to get a bit short with people and very much want to be left alone. Likely to burst into tears or tear someone's head off. Actually it's a very effective stage at work for pushing projects through and not taking anyone's shit.	Sometimes just felt so tired I could stay in bed for days – not sleeping (chronic insomnia) but just 'zoned out'. Valium wouldn't touch the sides. Waking at night, needing phantom wees. Two or three times a year it would be like a tsunami event and cause damage to my relationship. Tried to stay away from people and just wish the time away.
TREATMENT	Recently had a Mirena IUD fitted on recommendation by her doctor to manage the severity of her periods; the blood loss and emotional symptoms are still there but alleviated, and her iron levels are normal for the first time.	Took hormones from the age of 40 and then had her ovaries removed at 43, which gave her almost immediate peace.

CHAPTER 7

THE UNCOMFORTABLE
TRUTH ABOUT
ANXIETY

Yumi once had a panic attack on live TV. She was about to interview a footy player, and the only thing she found when she googled him was that he'd cheated on his wife. On air, Yumi said, 'I've read his autobiography, and amazingly it's not written in crayon!' – thinking she was very funny. Her boss came on to set with a thunderous look on her face to tell Yumi that the footy guy, who was watching from the green room, had complained about her joke.

In that moment Yumi's sense of safety plunged into a bottomless ravine. She'd just survived months of bullying in the mainstream media, receiving hundreds of death threats and copping some pretty wild social media abuse – all due to an earlier on-air gag about a *different* macho white guy. Now she felt it was all about to happen again. Her heart started pounding so hard she thought the sound of it must be coming through her mic. There was a deafening roar in her ears. She actually thought she was going to drop dead on the couch on national TV.

In the week before her first-year uni exams, Claudine was sitting on the floor of her friend's bedroom when her friend started reading out an incantation (essentially a magic spell – don't judge, it was the 90s) from a super creepy book. In that moment it was like a switch had been flipped. Claudine's heart started pounding. The hairs on the back of her neck stood on end. She broke out in a cold sweat. She thought she was going crazy.

Her friends didn't know what to do, so they took her to ... A PRIEST. He was very kind and tried to comfort Claudine with prayer, but he had no idea how to help. For what it's worth, that evening several people learnt that Hail Marys do not ease a panic attack.

Given that **one in three Australian women experiences anxiety at some point in their lives**, there's a pretty good chance that you have your own anxiety story. Anxiety is the most common mental illness in Australia – it affects one in four Australians and is more likely to affect women than men. Some figures suggest it's even more widespread. A 2020 survey from Jean Hailes found that one in two women between the ages of 18 and 24 reported having anxiety. The survey also found that anxiety was even more prevalent for First Nations women, women with disabilities and those who identified as LGBTQIA+.

Back in 2018, *Ladies, We Need To Talk* made a podcast episode about anxiety. We talked about the anxiety many of us experience as a sometimes-useful response that can keep you safe from danger. But when your fears are persistent and disproportionate to the threats you face, and this starts to interfere with your ability to live life, then you may have an anxiety disorder.

Since then, things have changed. (Cue deranged laughter.) Many of us find ourselves in circumstances where there are valid things to feel anxious about. We've had bushfires that destroyed homes and communities around the country, and produced smoke that spread even further. Cataclysmic evidence of climate change comes at us from the daily news and from the places where we live. We've had our lives upended by a pandemic, which returns like waves that knock us down any time we feel like we start to get back on our feet.

So it's fair to say we have reason to worry.

The thing is, these events are merely exposing a truth that has always been so: NOTHING IN LIFE IS CERTAIN, especially for those who are most vulnerable, including women. But there is help available, as well as treatments, skills and practices that can help us in uncertain and anxiety-provoking times.

Ladies, we need to talk about ANXIETY.

If you need someone to talk to, call:

Lifeline on 13 11 14
Suicide Call Back Service on 1300 659 467
Beyond Blue on 1300 22 4636
Headspace on 1800 650 890
QLife on 1800 184 527
Alcohol Drug Information Service
on 1800 250 015

THE MOST COMMON TYPES
OF ANXIETY DISORDER

Anxiety isn't one mental health condition – it's actually a group of conditions.

Generalised anxiety disorder is where you feel anxious most days and are constantly worried about a bunch of different things in a way that exceeds the level of threat they pose to your safety.

Panic disorder involves having recurrent, sudden and intense feelings of fear resulting in panic attacks (i.e. racing heart, breathing fast, sweating, thinking you are going to die). Panic disorder does not mean a one-off panic attack, but it can include the ongoing fear you will have a panic attack.

Social anxiety means that your intense fear of being awkward, criticised, embarrassed or humiliated in everyday social situations – such as making small talk or eating a meal – stops you from being able to connect with others.

Phobias involve an intense fear of a specific situation (e.g. being in an enclosed place – claustrophobia), activity (e.g. flying – aerophobia), or thing or object (e.g. spiders – arachnophobia). Being exposed to the phobia stimulus may cause a panic attack and/or prompt you going to extreme lengths to avoid it.

Then there are mental illnesses in which anxiety is a strong feature, but these are not technically grouped with anxiety.

Obsessive-compulsive disorder (OCD) involves repeating thoughts and behaviours over and over again to reduce intrusive thoughts or feelings of anxiety. An example is fear of germs and contamination, and excessively washing your hands as a way to ease this.

Post-traumatic stress disorder (PTSD) can happen after you experience a frightening event in which it felt like your life, or that of someone you love, was threatened, regardless of whether or not you were hurt. The event may be either witnessing or experiencing an accident, abuse, physical harm or a disaster. PTSD can involve involuntarily reliving the event, being hypervigilant, feeling emotionally numb or avoiding reminders of the event.

To feel anxious *can* be a very rational human response, and in certain situations it *can* give us a useful kick up the butt or keep us out of real danger. But when feelings of anxiety start to interfere with your daily life, then your anxiety is no longer serving you and it may start to meet the criteria for anxiety disorder.

Signs that you may need to see someone for some help managing your anxiety can show up as feelings (panicky, irritable, scared, worried or afraid most of the time, tense or on edge), thoughts ('I can't calm myself down', 'I might die', 'everything is going to go wrong') and physical sensations (sleep problems, excessive thirst, upset stomach, pins and needles, pounding heart, sweating). These are just some of the signs – for more, both Beyond Blue and Black Dog Institute have excellent user-friendly resources on their websites.

But why are some of us more prone to anxiety than others?

Anxiety has a few drivers and is rarely caused by a single thing. Family history and genetic pre-disposition lay down a crucial bedding in which anxiety can grow. Then there's early trauma and other life events, personality traits, coping styles, hormones and brain chemistry, and physical health. Also ... addictions? Yes. Unrelenting caring responsibilities? Yep. Financial pressure? For sure. Relationship stress? Doesn't help.

And why are women over-represented?

In 2016 a team of researchers from the University of Cambridge reviewed the global research into who is most affected by anxiety. From 48 high-quality studies, the researchers found **women were almost twice as likely to experience anxiety as men**. Some of the reasons for this include brain chemistry and hormonal changes across the lifespan. They also found that the way women react when faced with life challenges contributed to anxiety.

Anxiety can be linked with certain personality traits – such as perfectionism – or certain coping styles – such as ruminating or imposing rigid routines – that tend to be more common in women.

Cass Dunn, a clinical and coaching psychologist, says these are often a way of trying to create a sense of certainty in our lives and reduce the ambiguity that many of us struggle to live with. 'At the core of these behaviours is a very low tolerance for risk or uncertainty or ambiguity and a need, as best as they can, to plan and predict and control their world.'

Francis* is often paralysed by her perfectionism. 'The way I was brought up and my nature – you should be making the world a better place, you should be contributing to society. But if I can't do it perfectly, there is no point. I just don't do anything.' For instance, if she can't find what she believes to be the perfect birthday present, she won't buy anything at all. If she doesn't know exactly what to say in a text message, she doesn't respond. Then she feels terrible about herself for letting people down!

Francis says her dad often says he'd like both her mum and Francis to ease off a bit. 'At Christmas, he said, "I think we should all have the resolution to do less, care less and rest more." He is just content with whatever he is doing. My brothers are the same. It's the women who suffer from it in my family.'

Many of us believe that perfectionism is worth striving for, but Dunn says, 'It's really a deep fear of judgment or criticism or rejection or not feeling good enough.'

Even though anxiety is the most prevalent mental health condition in Australia, it's often treated as a less 'serious' issue. There are likely a few reasons for this, but one seems to be that you can have anxiety and still be highly productive. To the external world, it can look like you're busy juggling all the things. Sometimes we can't tell what's going on until something snaps or someone points it out.

Dunn says sometimes those who appear to be highly organised, meticulous, competent or capable can be wearing themselves out trying to maintain control. 'All of that behaviour is really underpinned by this fear that if they let go of any of that control then things will spin into chaos, and they do not have the capacity to cope with that.'

She believes we're all on a spectrum of being able to tolerate ambiguity and uncertainty, and those of us who really struggle with this tend to be more anxious. 'I think that a lot of people don't even necessarily twig that, "Oh. my perfectionism is actually a manifestation of anxiety." "Oh, the way I'm so rigid with my routines or my meal planning is actually a form of anxiety." "My imposter syndrome, the fact that I feel like nobody should have ever given me this job and I'm not good enough, and I don't belong or deserve to be there – that's just another manifestation of anxiety."'

Truth is, many of us are quite good at hiding our anxiety and making it seem as though everything is fine, and then we find that it overwhelms us and we can't keep it all inside.

Dunn says what sits beneath things like perfectionism is a massive amount of socialisation that starts when we're young girls. 'No matter how progressive we are as parents, they grow up in a world that reinforces that the girl's value is being nice and playing nice and being quiet and being polite and sharing.'

Could it be the actual reasons for anxiety are NOT ALL IN YOUR HEAD?

Could it be that there are some big menacing forces that can have a huge impact on our lives and we have no control over it? Maybe it's the caring work – both seen and unseen – that unequally falls to us? The gender discrimination that shows up as very serious issues like social and economic inequality and gender-based violence? The looming climate catastrophe? The fact that if you're Indigenous and incarcerated, there's a strong chance that you could be killed? Or the fact that the fastest rising rates of homelessness are among women over 55, according to a 2019 Australian Human Rights Commission report? Or that almost EVERY one of us has a story of sexual harassment or assault?

The World Health Organization (WHO) says **gender is a determining factor in poor health and mental illness** – including for anxiety.

There's no doubt that certain women experience more damaging gender inequality than others – First Nations women, women of colour, women with disabilities and members of the LGBTQIA+ community are disproportionately affected. As the WHO puts it: 'There is a positive relationship between the frequency and severity of such social factors and the frequency and severity of mental health problems in women.'

And all of this has been made SO much worse by the pandemic.

I was working in an office where I was the only woman in the building. Someone was really offended that there were tampons in the bathroom and was asking me, 'Are they yours? Why are they there?' And I got really upset. I felt like it was a sexist attack. It was a gay guy asking and I don't think he had sisters and I think it was a genuinely unusual thing for him to see tampons in the bathroom. We ended up having a really long back and forth about it and every word exchanged made me go deeper and deeper into this feeling of anxiety.

Then he wanted to discuss it again the next day! And at first I thought it was to apologise, but actually he wanted an explanation as to why the company would be wasting money paying for tampons. That whole thing sent me to a point where I was shaking, I was red in the face, my voice was trembling trying to have this conversation with this person. The conversation was enough to have me anxious in any circumstance, but I was already premenstrual and that made it so much worse. It's that stupid thing where you have to explain and you have to apologise, but he was the one being a dickhead! – **KELLIE**

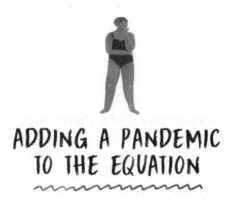

ADDING A PANDEMIC
TO THE EQUATION

It's often said that many women do the double shift: paid work at *work* and then unpaid caring work at home. Since the pandemic, it's been the TRIPLE shift: paid work, caring work and the mental load of worrying about it all.

We probably don't need to tell you this, but the pandemic has had a significant impact on women's lives and mental health. In late 2020 the Women's Mental Health Alliance published a report that showed how COVID restrictions in Victoria impacted on men and women differently, worsening existing structural inequalities. Turns out, we're not all in this together.

Here's a bit more on what they found in that report. It's difficult to read (there's a reason Yumi cried in the episode on this topic), but it's important to consider. Periods of crisis sometimes force things to the surface that would otherwise remain unnoticed, and this can be a catalyst for progress.

It's something to hold on to in these anxiety-inducing times. That, and the hands of the women in your life who give you courage, strength and love.

Women disproportionately represent those working on the COVID-19 frontline. They are more likely to be health and aged care workers, teachers, and social assistance workers. This means having to live with the stress of high work pressure AND the risk of infection. Small side note: much of the personal protective equipment (PPE) that is supposed to protect people while doing this work DOESN'T EVEN FIT women because it has been designed with men's sizes as the default.

The COVID-19 recession has been called a 'pink recession'. Australia's gender pay gap has widened due to COVID. More women have lost jobs than men, partly because many of the industries hardest hit by the lockdowns (and facing the longest recoveries) are female-dominated and also because women are more likely to be in lower-paid, insecure, part-time or casual roles, which were the first to go.

Women disproportionately bear the burden of caring responsibilities, including homeschooling, caring for family with disabilities and those living alone – even when they are still trying to hold down a job.

Lockdowns force women to stay home, even when home is unsafe. The 2020 survey found that one in four women experienced some form of intimate partner violence from a current or previous partner in the past 12 months. This intimate partner violence included emotional abuse, controlling behaviours, physical violence and sexual violence.

And for the most vulnerable women in our society it has been even worse. Women with pre-existing mental health conditions have become more unwell, migrant and refugee women have been more exposed to the risk of getting COVID and losing their jobs, and women with disabilities have lost access to vital health support networks and healthcare.

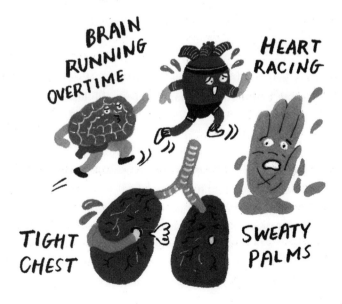

BRAIN RUNNING OVERTIME

HEART RACING

TIGHT CHEST

SWEATY PALMS

In the same way that many of us are being forced to live with ambiguity because of what is happening to and on our planet, there are times in our lives when we *have* to live with a certain amount of uncertainty.

The postnatal period is one time where a number of things can provide the perfect environment for anxiety.

For the person who carried and birthed the baby, hormones can have a huge influence on moods and mental health. It can be a *major* factor.

In the days after birth, oestrogen and progesterone levels fall off a cliff. It's common to have a strong emotional reaction (characterised by 'weepiness') on Day 3 after birth. In the weeks and months after that, you're likely to be dosing up on oxytocin, the 'bonding hormone', which, aside from making you feel wildly in love with your baby, can also make you vigilant for threats to said baby.

Hence, a bit of ... oh, anxiety.

Then there is all the shit – and by that, we mean literal shit – that comes with looking after an infant. Poo. Sleeplessness. The crying, the holding, the responsibility, the leaking body, the laundry!

Did we mention all the expectations that new mums face? We're expected to know how to parent small humans AND have a clean house AND be beatific AND consider having sex as if that's even faintly a good idea AND get back to our pre-pregnancy weight. Gross.

Not all of us will experience anxiety after having a baby, but it can be a pretty big trigger for many of us. 'That's a really good example of how suddenly all of those strategies stop working,' says Dunn, referring to the way we use routine and perfectionism to cope.

> 'When you have a major life change – something comes into your life that you can't control anymore and it all falls apart.'

My 10-month-old daughter has had every trouble sleeping under the sun. We live in an old block of flats, and my downstairs neighbour recently let me know that my child is keeping her up and that it's definitely due to my inability to parent properly (my very involved husband failed to get a mention, of course). Pretty small in the scheme of things right now, but with her words ringing in my ears every night, my anxiety has gone through the roof – something I've never really experienced before. – **STEPHANIE**

Another time when anxiety might surface is PERIMENOPAUSE.

In the lead-up to menopause, your hormones are completely all over the shop. This means you're getting hot flushes, erratic periods, and sleep inexplicably evades you.

Perimenopause also comes along, completely uninvited, at a time in many women's lives when they are dealing with a LOT. Demands coming from all sides – work, partners, kids, caring for older parents, a body that needs more looking after ...

Dunn says the expectations placed on women during this period can be fairly relentless.

'Many women in this age group have got kids in school and then ageing parents. The more things that you have to hold – whether it's COVID or homeschooling or something else – then you realise that you just can't continue to hold all that stuff; it just becomes too much. That's when you no longer have the capacity or the resources to manage the level of the demand.'

Yumi and Valaska have been friends for 15 years. For the past two, they've barely seen each other. The pandemic has kept them apart and Valaska has been flat out caring for her ailing parent.

'My mother was living with me and had a call bell that would ring night and day. Night and day. She couldn't even lift a cup to her mouth with her physical disability. It made me feel grumpy – a bit like when you've got a baby needing a feed every two hours. You love them and you nurture them but at the same time you feel a bit resentful. At least with a baby you know how long it will go for. You know there are phases that kids go through. But with my mother I didn't know how long it would last.'

The pressures on Val came from both directions. 'I have a 15-year-old teen with diagnosed anxiety who has not attended school since the end of primary school. I had hoped my mum would be a support at this time of my life but because of a physical disability she became like an infant in her body.'

And that's not all. Valaska herself has been managing her own health issues. 'I pretty much put myself on the back burner and I do have a bit of anxiety that there are lifestyle and stress factors that affect the chances of my cancer returning. I take hormone blocker medication every day to stop the cancer metastasizing. But there are other factors that could make the cancer return – high stress is a contributing factor, sedentary lifestyle, comfort eating processed foods and alcohol – all things I turn to to manage my stress and the opposite to what I'm meant to be doing!

'There is the niggling worry that the things I do to manage my anxiety will literally shorten my life.'

Berno is a solo mum who used to work hot jobs in the music industry but after a difficult divorce and relocation now works as the primary carer for her son who has autism, ADHD and anxiety.

'I feel like I'll always live on the edge of my nerves,' says Berno. 'My anxiety is daily and deeply manifested due to having to look after a little human on one income. I think about money constantly.'

The carer's pension she's on 'allows' her to work up to 20 hours per week – but it's near impossible to find a job between 9 am and 2 pm. Berno describes the fear of overfilling the car at the petrol bowser, or the guilt she feels when she lets her kid buy new Lego. 'It feels like hypervigilance. Like everything sounds louder, my jaw is always clenched, my shoulders are fused to my ears.

'There's a constant repetition of the "what if" always playing over worst-case scenarios. It can take just one big thing to destabilise everything. I wake at least a few times per week worrying about things like how to pay for new school shoes. I know money isn't the be all and end all, but fuck it helps!'

✳ ✳ ✳

A common refrain you hear from people who are anxious is something we've heard throughout the pandemic: 'I can't complain' or 'I know we're lucky so I shouldn't be upset'. It's OK to express our pain and our anxiety, especially when it comes with good reason. Others might have it worse, but misery is not a competition. Needing or wanting to howl at the moon, cry in the corner or march in the streets is completely reasonable.

Even without a global pandemic, anxiety would still exist. No matter what our (wildly uncertain) futures hold, even if it's 100 per cent roses, cuddles and a giant cushion of wealth (HA!), we're still going to need coping mechanisms.

If anxiety is affecting how you live your life then it's important to get help. The sooner, the better. Your GP is a good place to start, as are the helpline details back on page 107. Accessing professional help means you're a step closer to getting the kind of treatment or support that will work BEST FOR YOU.

One positive is that research suggests women are more likely to talk about mental health problems and seek help when struggling. (This may also explain why women are more represented in statistics.) It's much better to air what's worrying you than to bottle it up. Encourage discussion among friends and family, and remember that listening is as important as talking – make sure that whoever you're talking to about these issues feels heard as well.

Kellie (who we heard from earlier in the chapter) has learnt how to manage her condition. 'If I feel anxiety coming on, I just have to breathe. Knowing how to breathe deeply changes everything – changes your heartbeat, focuses your thoughts. I take a big deep breath in and in my mind say the word "slow" and breathe out and say the word "down". It works. It's like my "power down" button.'

Beth appeared in the anxiety episode of the podcast. She has found ways to alleviate her struggle with climate anxiety. 'If I'm feeling climate anxiety well up inside of me, I know that I need to go and spend some time with my children. I need to dance. Dancing is so powerful. Or I need to sing. I need to be in nature. I need to get my shoes off. Feel the ground beneath my feet. I have literally hugged trees.'

Sarah Wilson has written a book about anxiety and experiences it herself. She finds that what helps her is ACTION. 'Anxiety can be paralysing because our brains go into fight or flight – but when the problem is so large [like the climate crisis], we go into freeze mode. The best antidote for the overwhelm that we feel is action. Even if it's just being a really good recycler!'

Sarah found there are certain things that can really help when she is feeling anxious:

- ★ **Prioritise sleep, not short-term relief.** Sleep really is a big factor in your mental health and part of a long-term solution. Alcohol and other drugs can offer 'fast relief' for feelings of anxiety – but you will pay dearly for it later, plus they won't help you sleep. Looking after yourself sometimes means denying yourself the things that feel good but are actually treacherous for your mental health. Instead, do what you need to do – or avoid what you need to avoid – to get a good night's sleep.
- ★ **Follow the voices speaking truth to power.** You don't need to carry every burden in the world, but you can amplify the people who are fighting for justice. Do the work in learning about issues, live and breathe change, but remember, you don't have to be the instigator. Be part of a movement.
- ★ **Pause and be grateful.** It's such a corny thing to say but it does make a difference to remind yourself of the privilege, joy and good fortune

that have visited you. Yes, bad things happen to you – but so do good things. Gratitude helps to line up your values with your actions. 'It creates congruence in the brain, which creates an incredible sense of belonging and that all is right in the world,' says Sarah. 'It tells our nervous system that there's a natural order of things.'

★ **Disconnect and get outside.** There's a lot of bad news in the media and it can be difficult to tune out. But sometimes it's necessary to find spaces for joy and kindness. Self-care often means unplugging, switching the phone off and getting outside.

★ **Take a walk.** 'Walking triggers beta waves in the brain and tells our system that all is well, because if we're walking then we mustn't be under threat!' says Sarah. 'There's psychiatrists who do all their work while walking, and I wrote my books while walking.' Even when you're feeling lazy, just a 10-minute walk has significant benefits – immediately and in the long term. If you can't walk then try for some other physical activity.

Cass Dunn has something that she thinks we all need to add to this list. Based on her experience working as a clinical and coaching psych and speaking to experts and people with lived experience, she thinks there is one vitally important thing we all need to do when we're starting to feel anxious: SIT WITH IT.

'It's just learning to sit with anything that feels uncomfortable. To me, that's kind of my mission in life: to get people to learn to be able to manage a little bit of discomfort and not have to feel like they need to fix everything or solve it or improve it.'

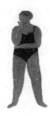

LET'S TALK ABOUT
BOOZE, BABY

Many of us turn to alcohol to rub off the rough edges of life's stresses. The truth is, alcohol makes anxiety worse – and you don't have to drink a lot for it to have an impact.

Researchers have been worried about women's drinking habits, especially those of middle-aged women, for some time. But the shitshow that is COVID-19 has seen women drinking more to cope with the stresses of lockdown, homeschooling, job loss and financial stress.

Even if your lockdown drinking feels like it is easing your stress and anxiety, it ultimately can leave you feeling *more* anxious.

While alcohol changes your brain chemistry and can have a sedating effect, when these effects wear off you can feel worse as your body processes the alcohol. Drinking alcohol to relieve anxiety can set up a vicious cycle where you drink to relax, this initially helps you feel calmer ... until the effects of the alcohol start to wear off and it leaves you feeling more anxious. Drink, sleep, remorse, repeat.

Doctors will often ask patients who present with anxiety about their alcohol consumption. But it can be tricky to meaningfully wade through the gigantic list of reasons we might be anxious in a 10-minute consultation. And if you're ashamed or a bit embarrassed about one potential cause, like you're quietly nursing a little drinking problem? Well, it's pretty easy to get the doctor to move on to the next question.

Yumi used to get anxious before social situations because she was worried she'd say something stupid. So she'd drink a lot – which was pretty much a way of guaranteeing she *would* say something stupid! Then she'd ruminate on her behaviour, feeling so awful that there was no way she could face the next social situation *without* drinking. The hangovers left her shaky, ashamed and very, very anxious. She knew things were bad when she started getting intense vertigo every time she drove over a bridge, imagining the car plunging through empty space.

Sarah's drinking and anxiety collided back when she was 26. 'It had tipped over from partying and drinking and that being my identity to actually being dependent on alcohol – having to have a drink to get rid of the shakes, drinking in the morning, and having to drink to function. I had been an anxious kid but it reached a new level as my drinking increased. I had been self-medicating – and then it stopped working.

'The severe anxiety manifested as being terrified to leave the house until I'd had sufficient alcohol – but even then it was still very difficult. I found it extremely hard to make phone calls and go to appointments. I avoided many social events. My relationships with family and friends became strained. Some of the worst symptoms were panic attacks and lying in bed for hours, unable to move.'

Yumi quit drinking more than four years ago and plans to never resume.

And Sarah?

'My life's completely different now. After many attempts to control my drinking – swapping this for that, knowing it was bad, thinking, "This is *not* good" – getting sober took about six years. I got lots of professional help, detoxed, rehabbing, and eventually I got sober. It's been seven years. I feel very fortunate that I have a really tight support network and that is so important. Connection with people is so important even though those relationships became strained. I definitely damaged a few relationships beyond repair, but my family and really close friends stayed with me.

'The anxiety was quite bad for a while – not having my "medication" (alcohol) – but it's basically non-existent now.'

Yumi says that like quitting smoking, quitting alcohol can take a few tries before it really sticks, but she thinks the best thing you can do is admit you have a problem. Once you do that, it's harder to be ashamed and you can start to fix it – with help. Talk to your GP, the Alcohol Drug Information Service or any of the other help lines on page 107.

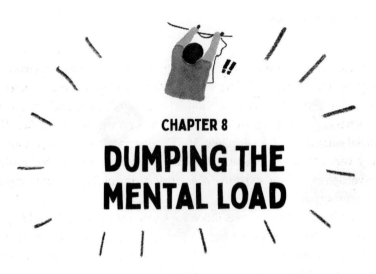

CHAPTER 8

DUMPING THE MENTAL LOAD

*H*ey, I have pre-ordered Avery's lunch and recess from the canteen on Friday, but he'll still need something for fruit break ... Can you please organise? If he's with you on Thursday and it's easier for me to order his lunch for then too, let me know and I can do it tonight as well.

Claudine's sister-in-law Edwina was one day away from HAVING A BABY when she sent that text. Between marking essays, washing clothes for a newborn and calling the hospital for an update on her induction, she was organising lunch for her kid. A lunch three days away!

Edwina, by the way, is not single. She's married to a man, a good man, the father of her children – and like many dads, he's considerate, competent and kind. But it's not *his* brain fizzing with lists and tasks while his wife prepares to deliver their baby.

You want to see what the mental load looks like? *That's it.* An endless mental list that you need to keep track of. ALONE. Even when you're about to push a human out of your vagina.

The mental load is INVISIBLE (no-one knows you're doing it) and ENDURING (it never, ever ends) and it has NO BOUNDARIES (you often do it while doing something else).

No-one thanks you for it. No-one even acknowledges you do it. But worst of all? No-one *pays* you for it.

Ladies, we need to talk about our MENTAL LOAD.

✳ ✳ ✳

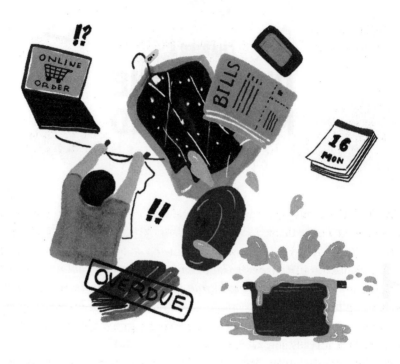

While we were making the very first episodes of *Ladies, We Need To Talk* back in 2017, a cartoon was going viral. It showed the French artist Emma visiting a friend's home for a meal. The friend is cooking dinner, feeding her two small children, trying to make conversation ... while her male partner sits down and chats to the artist over a drink.

When a pot overflows, Emma's exhausted friend loses it. The hapless partner is confused. 'You should've asked! I would've helped!' he cries.

What made so many of us hit 'like/share' was that Emma had given shape, and a name, to the list-making, box-ticking and task-delegating that occupies so much of our headspace. Emma had created a scene that those of us living in heterosexual relationships know well.

Emma had drawn the mental load.

MENTAL LOAD

The invisible, intangible work you do inside your head to keep your household running and the people you love alive, fed, clean, healthy, happy and safe.

Any of the following sound familiar?

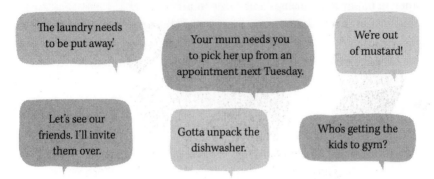

It's well documented that when men and women live together, women do the bulk of the domestic labour – and this did not change in the lockdowns of 2020 and 2021, when most of us were at home *all* of the time. In fact, a bunch of research has found it made the situation worse.

Carrying the mental load is not just about doing all of the actual work. It's about being the person who is responsible for making sure things happen. And they're often little things – like lunches. Not a big deal, but if it's forgotten? Someone little literally goes hungry!

In the domestic space, the mental load is a burden unevenly skewed towards women. WE RUN THE HOUSE! We're also the head of tending relationships. Fridge-stocker and logistics lead. CEO of keeping everyone healthy. Chief 'find my socks' officer. This is not a fleeting part of a work week – it's every. Single. Day. Then there's the extra seasonal load that we pick up with birthdays, anniversaries, family reunions and … Christmas.

In Yumi's family, the women get to work planning Christmas in *October*. They organise gifts. They know everyone's favourite foods and allergies. They know freezer space and oven dimensions. They have contingencies arranged for unexpected guests, bad weather, an emergency hip replacement.

On December 25, the men show up holding a bottle. (And let's be real, they probably didn't even buy the bottle.) They then sit around eating and drinking, maybe play a bit of cricket with the kids, maybe ineffectively prod at a sausage with some tongs, while the women of all generations prep and serve and clean and spread cheer AT A SPRINT. Merry fucking Christmas.

After the mental load episode of *Ladies, We Need To Talk* went to air, we heard from many women who were first learning about the mental load from the podcast. We heard from older women and younger women. We heard from women who had tiny babies and others with adult children. There were women in happy relationships and single mums.

They were all relieved to know they weren't the only ones going to bed at night with their brains fizzing. What they all had in common was the same sense of outrage that makes us want to burn shit to the ground.

> I cannot thank you enough for your episode on the mental load ... it has helped me SO much to know I'm not alone in struggling with this. – **CLAIRE**

> Thank you for reminding me ... I am, in fact, NORMAL. And not just a cranky mum. – **HELEN**

> Your podcast brought to the brim all these hidden, invisible responsibilities we shelve in the bursting filing cabinets of our minds. Not just remembering the birthday presents we need to buy, the tradesmen to call and the school fees to pay, but the emotional wellbeing of the introvert who doesn't say much or the normally bouncy daughter who is so completely crushed when someone excludes her at school. Add to that the friend who is struggling through a divorce or illness. A recently widowed mother. A sister with a challenging child. And an untoned stomach that needs to be reintroduced to 'engaging my core', and my brain becomes an impossible weight to lug around. – **KYLIE**

The mental load is something that can affect all women – regardless of the load they might already be carrying in their lives and careers, and the structures they might have in place to try to keep things even at home.

Journalist and author Tracey Spicer had a lightbulb moment about how the mental load was showing up in her life, even though she and her partner equally share the housework and childcare.

'It was just the little things. Like, I'm always the one who organises school holiday care. Or who takes the time off to look after the kids if they're sick. Or arranges everyone's Christmas presents or birthday presents in his extended family and my extended family.'

NSW Greens MP Jenny Leong had a similar sense of recognition, which was quickly followed by panic.

'I was like, "Oh, no! Now I've added that to my mental load", thinking about how often I think about the mental load!'

The thing about the mental load is that it's pretty much invisible until you know what to look for.

Harvard University sociologist Allison Daminger found that the mental load can be broken down into four parts. Let's use our earlier canteen/getting-ready-to-have-a-baby scenario with Edwina as an example.

1. **Anticipating the job that needs doing** (*Our kid will need lunch on Friday – while I'm having a baby.*)
2. **Making the decision** (*I will order him a canteen lunch.*)
3. **Instructing others** (*I'll text Claudine to make sure he gets the canteen lunch.*)
4. **Monitoring** (*I'll follow up to make sure lunch was had – oh, did I mention I am HAVING A BABY?*)

Overwhelmingly, the anticipation and monitoring parts fall to women, and men step up for the decision-making.

Associate Professor of Sociology at the University of Melbourne Leah Ruppanner spends her time researching and writing about gender inequality, including domestic labour and the mental load. She points out that 'ALL people have a mental load – men AND women. Some portion of your mental load may go to thinking about your career. Some portion of it may go to thinking about your family. Some portion of it may go to thinking about your personal life.'

The difference is what men and women are thinking *about*.

'Men are spending a lot more of their mental load thinking, "How do I advance my career?" They're using their brain power thinking about the day-to-day challenges of work. Women might be thinking about work and career advancement, but they're also thinking, "Who's going to pick up the child from day care?" or "What are we doing for school holidays?" or "Who's doing the housework?"'

One of these will lead to better financial security and personal growth, and the other …? Not so much! No wonder women face greater financial instability as they get older.

Dr Ruppanner also points out that there is a difference in how we divide up domestic labour and the mental load that comes with those tasks. 'Routine tasks tend to be done by women. These are things that require immediate attention – cooking, changing nappies, cleaning, doing the laundry. These jobs need to be done regularly … usually multiple times a day.

'Men tend to do non-routine or episodic chores – taking out the rubbish, changing a lightbulb, mowing the lawn.'

And while those jobs have the image of being technical or 'manly' – the truth is they take a lot LESS cumulative time than those multiple-times-a-day jobs that women get. Taking out the bins? Probably less than three minutes every week. Cooking dinner? Around an hour PER DAY.

It's pretty clear what we lose when our brain space and energy are sucked up by the mental load:

- ★ You're probably not thinking as much about your paid labour and how to set yourself up for a financially stable future.
- ★ You're probably not thinking about what you need to do to stay physically and mentally healthy.
- ★ You're probably not getting enough sleep, which is just bad news all round.
- ★ You're probably getting the utter shits with your partner.

While each woman's experience of the mental load is unique, most are able to pinpoint the moment when it grows exponentially – when the *kids* arrive.

'Once people marry, women start doing more, men do less, and once they have babies, everybody's housework goes up … but the gap widens again,' says Dr Ruppanner.

Jenny Leong certainly found this when she had her first child and then returned to her work as a politician. 'The mental load of breastfeeding is insane, because actually there are physical ramifications if you don't remember to pump or feed at the right times. I was spending a lot of time sitting in meetings going, "OK, now I've got five minutes between that meeting and that thing and there's going to be a vote in parliament at that time. I need to be able to take my top off to do my pumping."'

When Jenny's partner went back to work after his paid parental leave, she noticed the mental load burden shift again. 'Once we were both back at work, the default position falls back to gender roles, and the expectation of who's supposed to know those things like birthdays and family events falls to me!

'Then you feel like, "Oh god, if I *do* this domestic stuff, am I being a bad feminist?"'

✳ ✳ ✳

Once we find ourselves carrying the mental load, it feels tricky to navigate out of it. Especially because, as we know from Emma's cartoon, a partner might say, 'Let me know if you need help' and think they're being generous.

But what they're really saying is, 'The mental load is yours and I refuse to take on a share.'

'LET ME KNOW IF YOU NEED HELP'
= 'EAT A SHIT SANDWICH'

The pattern seems to be: See the work. Delegate it to partner. Monitor situation (meaning it remains your mental load). Follow up. At this point the task is either completed, completed poorly (so you are back at the start), or vetoed (partner has deemed the task unworthy or unnecessary and thus refuses to do it). The lag between assignation and veto creates a tense line, expressed in the forehead wrinkles of the assigner.

So, how did we get to this point?

The patriarchy, of course. It's how we're raised from the moment we start playing house with dolls instead of breaking dump trucks. It's also what we see happening in front of us – generations of women doing this invisible work. So when we grow up, we do the same.

Tracey Spicer noticed her daughter, Grace, started taking on some of the family's mental load before she was 10. 'If someone's forgotten something in the house, she'll remember it. She'll know where the keys are. She'll know when we have to go shopping.

'She's looked around her in society and thought, "I have to be able to do everything to make it in this world."'

What's just as interesting is what was happening with Tracey's son. 'I don't know whether as a result of that, or if it happened before, but our son's become quite lazy to the point where he said a while ago, "When I move out of home, I don't need to learn to cook because Grace will cook for me!"'

Like Grace, many of us started taking on the mental load when we should have been playing soccer or climbing trees. From a young age, girls are encouraged to make life easier, nicer and more comfortable for everyone around them. It's a habit that sticks.

But that doesn't mean it is a habit we can't break.

Dr Ruppanner says it's important to think about the habits you develop when you go into a relationship. Don't 'play house' if you move in with a partner unless you want to continue doing his washing and reminding him to call his mother on her birthday.

She also says we need to ask ourselves about our role as gatekeepers of responsibility in the home. Why the bloody hell do we keep stepping in and taking on the responsibility?

'Is the concern that if men actually do the job they won't do as good of a job as the women would do? If that is the issue then we, as women, need to stop that.'

Or are we concerned that if we don't continue to remember and delegate all the things that need to be done, then they won't get done at all?

Dr Imaan Joshi is a doctor and single mum of four kids (aged 10, 12, 14 and 15) who's also running her own skin clinic. Her life is HECTIC.

We first met Dr Joshi when we made the mental load podcast episode and wanted to know more about what it looks like for a very busy working single mother. There is the undeniable load that goes with being the only person responsible for her four kids, but she actually found her burden *easing* after her marriage ended.

'I found it was a lot easier, because I no longer had to spend time, energy and effort to try and manage someone who, in some ways, had checked out of the marriage. I stopped expecting something.

'But it was also hard because I don't have anyone to share the kids' achievements with. I don't have anyone who is as invested in the kids as I am. I really miss that aspect of it. Having someone to sit down with at the end of the day, after the kids are in bed, and know that this is someone who's got my back just like I've got his back.'

We caught up with Dr Joshi again as we were writing this book, and since we last spoke her life has become even busier ... but even easier. Why? She's raised her children to be self-sufficient, capable humans. Humans who take on the full responsibility of certain tasks.

Chores are shared by all members of the household in an age-appropriate fashion. The older kids look after their younger siblings and make sure they get home from school safely and do their homework. Each member of the family makes dinner at least once a week – one of the kids cooks three nights a week!

'I said to them that everyone has to pick one day where they will cook dinner and one day where they will clean the kitchen. I don't care how simple it is – it can be a one-pot pasta dish. The oldest said, "I will teach the baby and supervise her to cook." The kids will text me and say, "Tell us when you are 15 minutes away. We've got dinner for you and we'll warm it up when you get home."'

Dr Joshi didn't ask her kids to *help* her with individual tasks or jobs – she delegated full responsibility for those things. This means those things are no longer taking up her brain space.

It also means she is no longer able to control exactly how the tasks are done. Her kids do the washing their way or make the dinner they want to make. If the towels aren't all folded the way she'd do them, that's cool.

But she's found when she makes this point to others, the conversation gets a little strained. 'I have conversations with women where I say to them, "You want it done the way you want it done. You don't want anyone else to do it because it's not good enough for you. In the process you're actually teaching people to leave it all to you."'

In same-sex couples the labour of the mental load can't fall to male–female roles, so it's usually negotiated according to skill and enthusiasm.

Clio and Jess have one daughter. 'Clio usually doesn't like being seen as "the dad" – unless it's to reference *Bluey*,' says Jess. 'Clio does more hours (9–5) and has a good paying job. This allows me more freedom to take work when I want, to be the pick-up, drop-off and afterschool mum, or look for other investment opportunities.

'I'm the bill payer, the decider of dinner and food, the one who is constantly booking trips – and yes, the birthdays, Santa and tooth fairy jobs all go to me. But she appreciates it all a lot – and I do love it ... THE SECOND Clio knocks off (paid) work, I "knock off" and Clio is "the go-to mum" … and seeing we purposely put Adia to bed at 10 pm because we are morning sleepers, it's hardly only the "dinner and kids straight to bed routine" that so many working parents get. Because of that I don't think Adia has a favourite mum.

'We flipped a coin and I got Father's Day and Clio gets Mother's Day. But seriously? We constantly check in on our "happy-ometer". I'm happy and she's happy.'

✳ ✳ ✳

Anyone who's ever seen a therapist will know that once you name something, it becomes easier to see, easier to air out, easier to SOLVE.

Here, we've called this idea the mental load, but it's also known as the 'second shift' and 'invisible work'. Eve Rodsky – author, Harvard-trained lawyer, mother of three and daughter of a single parent – likes 'invisible work' because a modicum of solution is offered in the name.

'I kept thinking, maybe if I could make VISIBLE all the invisible things I was doing for my home and family for my husband, Seth, maybe then he would value what I did,' says Rodsky. 'What I realised was that a lot of this *is* invisible work that's happening behind the scenes, which our partners don't know about.'

Rodsky says that in her hundreds of interviews with men, 'the number one thing men told me they didn't like about home life was "nagging". It was feeling like they couldn't do anything right.' And she attributes this to what she calls 'RAT': the Random Assignment of a Task.

'Men want to know their role,' says Rodsky. 'Men are being RAT-fucked all over the place.'

She says we need to approach this invisible work like how we do our *actual* work. 'Look at it like a business, like your organisation, like your workplace, where OWNERSHIP wins.'

In a business, you don't delegate – you give ownership of the whole thing. Delegation is a short-term solution. Ownership is a long-term solution. 'Imagine walking into your job today

NAGGING

Constantly harassing someone to do something. 'I wanted to get away from my nagging wife.' Similar: complaining, criticising, grumbling, fault-finding, moaning.

NAGGING (ALTERNATIVE USE)

Trying to delegate tasks to a person who refuses to take their share of a burden. 'I'd asked repeatedly for him to cook dinner just once a week and he accused me of nagging.'

and just saying to your producers, "Hey, so what should I be talking about today? I'll wait for you to tell me what to do." That kind of attitude just doesn't stand up in a workplace!

'But in our homes, we treat the crucial tasks with no respect, with no rigour ... Actually, the men who take ownership ... are reporting being happier in their home and they're willing to take on more.'

Once Yumi had been given the term 'mental load', she was able to use it in her relationship as a tangible way of dividing the invisible work. Her partner would ask, 'What's happening with the kids' lunches?' And she would say, 'Why are you giving me this mental load? It's a question you're capable of answering!' Or he'd say, 'Can we organise a space to put all the XYZ?' And she would say, 'I don't want that mental load. You organise the space and then tell me where it is.'

Yumi also gave her partner ownership over particular tasks by saying things like, 'I don't want to take the mental load of kids' doctor's appointments. Can you just have the numbers in your phone and make that your thing?'

Rhiannon was one of the many women who wrote to us about the mental load after hearing the podcast. 'At first I was like, "Pshhhh ... that doesn't apply to me." I'm like 23, I ain't about that life.'

A few months later, she'd just moved house and was doing the washing up and ran out of space to put the clean dishes. 'I frantically asked the bf to grab a tea towel and help dry, and he responded, "And the tea towels are ...?"'

Rhiannon wrote that something inside her snapped – 'I didn't know where my fucking clean undies were, much less the tea towels.' She says, 'He probably didn't deserve my short response, but I didn't appreciate the way he phrased his question. We both live in the same place. Why was it *my* responsibility to know the location of the tea towels?

'This episode really helped me decide to not put up with this shit. I ain't letting it creep in slowly now, only to find myself wading in it in 10 years!'

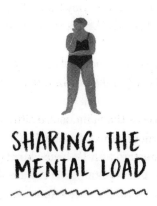

SHARING THE
MENTAL LOAD

Explicitly naming ALL the domestic work that women are burdened with means it can no longer be treated as invisible and may even be – *gasp!* – fairly distributed!

Eve Rodsky created a game called Fair Play that divides household work, visible and invisible, into a shareable, tangible deck of cards. There are 100 of them! But Rodsky warns: 'If you treat it like a list, like "you take dishes and I'll take garbage", it will never work. Consciousness raising without a solution is more harmful than not being conscious at all.'

Rodsky's solution lies in a framework she's called CPE: conception, planning, execution. To understand it, let's turn our thoughts to … mustard.

1. **Conception**: Somebody in your home has to know your youngest son likes yellow mustard on his sausages.
2. **Planning:** Somebody has to notice when that mustard's running low and put it on a grocery list.
3. **Execution:** Somebody has to get their butt to the store to purchase the mustard.

Rodsky's research has found that *execution* is where men step in. They don't do the first two tasks, but are asked to complete the third. They're sent to the shops to buy the mustard and that's a big problem because they bring home spicy Dijon when you wanted yellow mustard.

Then you have men everywhere saying things like, 'I can't even bring home the right type of mustard! My wife's yelling at me over mustard, so I'm not going back to the store for her!'

And women are saying, 'How can I trust my husband with things as important as our will, if I can't even trust him to bring home the right type of mustard?'

But when somebody owns the full mustard situation, from conception to planning to execution, when someone OWNS THE GROCERY CARD, then they know what type of mustard to get – because they have a context.

Apply CPE to any task. If one person is in charge of all three – conception, planning and execution – that's ownership! Ding ding! If not, have a conversation about it and make sure someone owns the card.

Reminder: There are 100 cards in Rodsky's Fair Play deck! That's a lot of conversations to have – including about tasks that you maybe haven't even thought of. The payoff will be worth it.

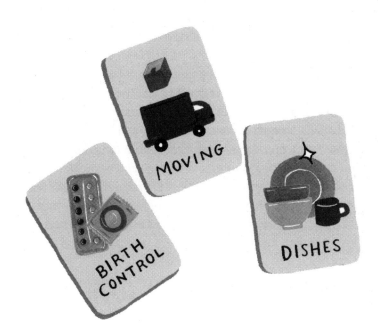

CHAPTER 9
THE POWER OF 'NO'

Would you like a bath? No. *Please put your shoes on.* Nope. *Could you eat this delicious meal that you didn't have to prepare or pay for?* Nuh-uh. *Could you ...?* Nnnnnnnnnooooooooooooooooooooooooooooooooo!

If you've ever spent time with a toddler, you'll know that humans are born with an inherent ability to say no.

But somewhere between being the three-year-old who screams in refusal while boldly throwing herself to the ground and the person we are when we finish school, we go backwards and *unlearn* how to say no.

'From childhood, women are socialised to make themselves likeable above everything else,' says writer, commentator and reforming people-pleaser Jamila Rizvi. 'If you talk to a little girl or even a teenage girl, being *liked* is generally number one on their list of aims in life. They want boys to like them. They want their friends to like them. They want parents and teachers to like them.

'I'm all for being a pleasant, friendly person. But we do socialise our girls so that when they find themselves saying no or pushing back on what they're asked for later in life, it feels like they're being bad.'

So here we are, again and again agreeing to situations we regret, and doing work we don't have time for that has no benefit to us and drains us of energy.

We've already established last chapter that anxiety is an issue for many women. But how's this? Research from Jean Hailes Women's Health Survey in 2018 found that **close to three quarters of women surveyed feel nervous or on edge nearly every day**.

There are a bunch of reasons for the levels of stress and anxiety in women's lives. But one thing we frequently hear from the *Ladies* community is that they just don't have enough time. The Jean Hailes research revealed that one-third of women don't get ANY time to themselves during the week.

This is where saying no comes in. It's not being selfish, it's about surviving. It's about taking care of yourself so you can say yes to the things that you *need* to do – work, look after others, stay well, stay sane, fight the patriarchy.

But for many of us, saying no is bloody hard. What are you going to do? Be the asshole who refuses to host Christmas? Absolutely abscond from homeschooling? Decline to throw that birthday party? Lie down on the floor and wail?

Ladies, we need to talk about SAYING NO.

✳ ✳ ✳

'Hey Yumi, do you mind preparing a salad for our picnic? I know you're so good at salads and love cooking!'
'Sure! How many people?'
'Twenty.'
'Oh. Wow.'

Sarah Knight has made a career out of encouraging people to say no.

Knight was in her 30s and working in publishing in New York when she hit a wall. 'I was having panic attacks in the office. I had terrible anxiety, which turned into depression.'

When she started peeling back the layers, trying to figure out what it was that was making her unwell, she realised she was trying to fit into a 'vanilla corporate structure' to which she was profoundly unsuited.

'Working in a professional environment and being a woman, I really felt like I had to put a lot of time, energy and money into my appearance. My clothes, my handbags, my make-up, blow-drying my hair, wearing heels to work. And then I finally realised, "What am I doing? I am spending an extra 45 minutes every day on something that I don't personally care about!" This was where so much friction was being created inside my brain and then inside my body.'

It was at that point that she knew things had to change. It wasn't just day-to-day stresses that could be appeased by leaving work early or getting a massage. Knight knew she needed to make big changes to her life. She started by saying no to things.

She said no to colleagues. She said no to family. She said no to friends. She said no to work requests, like unnecessary conferences, infinite email chains and long commutes to work. She said no to expectations she set for herself, like needing to look and dress the part. Ultimately, she said no to that vanilla corporate structure. She now works for herself and has written five self-help books on this topic.

'I am more mentally healthy than I have ever been. I am not perfect. There's a lot going on in the world right now, between politics and climate crisis and coronavirus, that are definitely giving me a run for my money.

'But I focus on the things I can do that are going to make me happier or that are going to mitigate my annoyance. I know there are things I have to do that maybe I don't really *want* to do, but I'm going to do them in the best way that works for me.'

Knight argues that we need to be thrifty with our most precious resources: time, energy and money. Much is made about the importance of being thrifty with our money. But Knight argues we shouldn't waste *any* of our resources, least of all TIME, which is the most finite. 'A lot of us have a sense of what's in our bank account, or at least in our wallet, at all times. Do the same for your time and energy and really visualise that when you spend it.'

She suggests thinking of your time, energy and money as 'fuck bucks'. Spend fuck bucks on things in your life *only if* you give a fuck about them. This is key.

What works for Knight (and many of the people who've bought her self-help books) is to treat fuck bucks as you would actual dollars. They are genuinely valuable. She considers the 'fuck budget' as the 'single best tool to decide whether something is worth your time, energy and money. That unlocks the door to sorting your "discard" pile of stuff that you don't care about – and that you don't want to give your time, energy and money to – from the stuff that you do.'

Of course there will be things that we cannot say no to, and for each one of us that list will look a little different.

If you have babies or small children, you will still need to feed them and change their nappies (BORING), but you probably don't have to make their goddamn pizza dough or handwash their clothes!

At work you might still need to go to meetings or make small talk with customers or answer emails, but you don't have to organise morning teas or go to team drinks. And you absolutely DO NOT have to do other people's dishes in the work kitchen!

Things that Yumi gives ZERO fuck bucks allocation:	Kicked off Claudine's give-a-fuck list:
★ men-only sports	★ complicated school lunches
★ opinions of strangers	★ school parents' committee
★ people who make her feel bad about the world	★ kids' sport (but will do choir, plays, debating and hiking)
★ school reports	★ cakes that require more than one bowl
★ work Christmas party	
★ making my own gyoza	★ washing floors
★ ironing	★ ironing

If you really sit and think about your 'fuck bucks', you might be surprised by what you find you can simply stop doing. One of the delightful things Knight has learnt is that 'there really aren't as many consequences as we think there are for saying no and setting boundaries and just being your authentic self'.

✳ ✳ ✳

'Hey Claudine, are you happy if you guys get the back room when we go away for Christmas?'
'Ahh ... you mean the one with bunk beds for all the kids?'

OK, so understanding that your time and energy are finite is crucial in our learning to say no.

But what about the actual ... *saying no* bit? How do we get the *words* to come out of our mouths? And *what* words, exactly? Is it really possible to say no without burning every bridge we've built and making everyone hate us?

Rachel Green is an emotional intelligence coach who teaches people how to identify and understand their emotions so they can manage them better. She argues that too often we let our emotions run the show.

The big emotion she helps many women with is GUILT. 'They feel guilty about saying no and therefore they give in and say yes.'

The guilt itself isn't an issue. It's the guilt-making-us-feel-like-we-have-to-say-yes bit that is. And the first step to freeing yourself of this guilt is to know when it is driving your decisions.

For instance, let's say your nephew is having a birthday party and you don't want to go. But this makes you feel like a bad sister and a bad aunt. You feel guilty. Instead of simply saying to your sister, 'I love you, but no,' you offer a complicated excuse involving a GP appointment, important shopping and a visit to a sick friend.

The problem is you have now given your sister (who means well, but wants you there to see her two-year-old blow out candles on a Saturday morning) a bunch of different problems to solve for you. To put it another way, you've opened yourself up to *negotiation*. 'Go see my GP – I checked for you, she has a spot this afternoon! Can you do the shopping later? And if you want, I can visit Sick Friend with you on Sunday!'

Now there's a strong chance that, come early Saturday morning, you'll be eating honey joys and wiping cupcake off the sole of your shoe before you can say 'hip hip hooray'.

The trick, Green says, is to notice your guilt at the outset and just sit with it. Don't offer excuses, and don't give in to it.

'We feel guilty simply because we have been trained to be nice. That's when we go, "No, this is just my training. I'm not actually doing anything wrong. Therefore, it's OK for me to say no. It's OK for me to stay guilty. But I don't have to give in to the guilt."'

Green has her own example of how adding excuses and justifications to your 'no' can backfire on you. 'We were sitting around one day in the staff-room and the boss said to us, "I need someone to go on a committee. There aren't many women on campus. We must have a woman representing us on the committee."'

When her boss asked her other colleagues if they could help out, they all simply said, 'No, I can't,' and that was that. Green, who was 27 at the time, had zero interest in being on another committee, so she told her boss, 'No, I'm sorry. I can't. I'm too busy.'

'She looked at me and fixed me in the eyes and said, "We're *all* busy, Rachel. You're going." I was the only one that added a reason and she was able to undermine and get rid of my reasoning.'

That's when she learnt. DO NOT JUSTIFY your behaviour. 'Just make a statement. "No, thank you." "No, I'm sorry, I can't do that."'

Sarah Knight agrees that making excuses or justifying your choices gives people an opportunity to argue with you. Her advice? Keep it simple.

'I know it feels unnatural to just say, "No, thank you," but it really is the best way to get started. Most people will say, "OK," and leave it at that. If they say,

"Oh, that's too bad. Are you sure you can't make it?" You can say, "Yeah, I know, but I really can't." That ends the conversation.'

MINDBLOWING!

If it doesn't end the conversation, Knight says you need to be firm: 'I've said no, and I really mean it. I hope you'll accept it. If you can't, I think that says more about you than it does about me.' Otherwise you might need to accept this person is not really someone you want to have a relationship with.

Another great suggestion of hers is the 'no-and-switch'.

Let's try the no-and-switch for your nephew's birthday party. Your sister asks you to come along and you say, 'No, I'm sorry I can't come to the birthday party, but how about we catch up for pizza on Tuesday night?'

Cue wild applause. You get to see your sister – on your own terms. No annoying party, no ruptured relationship.

For many of us, being assertive will feel uncomfortable and we're afraid of coming off as being blunt, cold or heartless. But there is an art to uttering that glorious 'no' without being rude – and that is an ART that can be learnt.

Green suggests always being polite and thanking people for asking you. 'Keep your voice pleasant because some women, when they're trying hard to maintain their boundaries and say no, often start to sound sarcastic or really arch.'

She also suggests you could give some context around your decisions to put boundaries in place, especially for those you are closest to who might find your 'no' hard to hear at first. This is not the same as offering an excuse for saying no, but about being clear on why you want to put boundaries in place.

Here are our top tips on how to say no:

★ Train your 'no' like a muscle. It might feel awkward at first, but it will get stronger.
★ Don't make excuses. Just give a clear, direct and very polite no.
★ Have set phrases up your sleeve.
★ Ignore your guilt. Ask yourself if your 'yes' will bring joy and delight.
★ Imagine what your life will look like if you say yes. (You at your nephew's birthday party, first thing on a Saturday morning, surrounded by a dozen screaming kids, brightly coloured food, so much noise ... Are you glad you capitulated?)
★ Remember your obligations are often self-imposed, not real.
★ Don't let the panic make you blurt bad words or excuses. You can still be polite, kind, firm AND say no.

My marriage therapist recently told me and my husband that because I've so repressed my ability to say no, I had to rediscover my inner two-year-old and say no, full stop, to whatever I wanted to. No apologies, no explanation, no 'no-and-switch' (although I find the no-and-switch a useful skill in everyday life with friends, work, etc.). So I had to get used to saying no to him without apology, and he had to get used to hearing no from me. A very liberating experience! – **ALLISON**

✳ ✳ ✳

To take this one step further, it is important to ACTIVELY try to create time in your life that is just for you. Sometimes that involves saying no to *yourself.*

When you talk to women who have clear boundaries, you soon learn that these feelings of guilt and obligation are often of our own making. Sometimes it takes a big life adjustment for people to realise this and start putting up their own boundaries, but it shouldn't have to be like that.

Dr Imaan Joshi, the busy single mum of four who we met in the previous chapter, carries very little mental load these days because she's learnt how to have boundaries – at home, in her friendships and especially at work.

'If the patient says, "I can't make it until 2 pm," but the clinic closes at one on a Saturday, I've had staff say, "That's OK, I'll stay back." I will say, "No, you won't. They can decide for themselves if this is important enough for them to move things around, or they're not going to attend. But why do you need to stay that extra hour?"

'As a doctor, it's really important when I'm in a consultation that I'm patient-centred and patient-focused. Doctors really aren't taught how to have boundaries and we're not taught how to show them. We're really not taught how to have a good conversation around difficult things.'

Dr Joshi decided to stop saying yes to things she didn't want to do because she noticed there was a loop. 'I'd say yes when I really wanted to say no but I kind of felt like I couldn't really say no. Then repeatedly, I felt angry, mad, resentful and annoyed.'

For Dr Joshi this period of reflection and personal growth was vital, not only because she was a doctor and raising four kids on her own, but also because her marriage had been abusive and she had patterns of behaviour she wanted to change. 'Often times in abusive relationships, the only way you're going to get along is by going along. So over time, because you're trapped, you make yourself agreeable to everything. But then it kind of bleeds into other aspects of your life as well.'

Jamila Rizvi had to make radical changes to her life after she got sick, really sick – and then stayed sick. 'Now I have a whole lot of disabilities that slow me down. I just had to relearn what my body is capable of.'

Rizvi uses her diary to block out time for herself, but it hasn't been easy for her. 'I am an extrovert and will always want to do more work, see more friends, hang out with people, be part of my community, but my body doesn't want me to do that. I've had to learn to say no to *myself*. I don't want to pretend that I have got there. I haven't. But I am slowly learning to be better at just deciding that I don't care enough about other people's opinions of me.

'There's nothing wrong with wanting to be pleasant to people, with wanting to be a warm and kind and generous person. But the reality is we will never please everyone. We will never be universally popular. And, actually, that's OK.'

It's OK. Let's sit with that for a minute.

It feels risky to admit it, but becoming happy with (and clever about) doing a 'good enough' job at work for the last few years, and not putting pressure on myself to be outstanding has had the biggest positive impact on my mental health. More surprisingly to me, it has had zero negative impact on my career. (I should say that my white middle-class privilege is obviously key to being able to get away with this choice.)

Work was getting out of hand so in order to do less (and also help my team do less), I made a decision to become a bottleneck. So nothing gets answered in under 24 hours. Miraculously, by the time you get round to answering it, someone else has often taken care of it. There's obviously urgent stuff, but I have also decided to take the time to call up and chat through any issues on the phone rather than generate more emails. It takes longer, which also has the effect of slowing everything down.

The upshot is, of course, that some things get missed. There's literally not enough time in the day to get through everything that's thrown at me. So I've become relaxed about the concept of some things just not getting done, or getting forgotten until someone reminds me, and it turns out that this is not much of a big deal. I reckon about a third of the stuff that I forget/ignore has also been forgotten by the person who asks me. – **KATE**

Not sure about you, but we've learnt something here. When you say 'no', the ground WILL NOT open up and swallow you. Pretty much everyone we've spoken to for this chapter agrees that once you start saying no, it's surprising how *few* people are upset by your response.

Rachel Green has another story about saying no at work.

'I was really scared that if I said no to this offer, it would be a career-limiting move. I practised and noticed I kept feeling guilty. So I decided to approach it as an experiment. I had this impression in my mind that if I felt guilty, and if I *disobeyed* the guilt, something dreadful would happen. Some hand would appear and slap me or this person would never talk to me again.

'So one day I stood in my office and this person asked me to do this thing. I stood there and I felt terribly guilty. I thought, "I am just going to stand here and feel guilty and … *very nicely say no!*"'

And guess what? Did the ground swallow her up? The sky fall in? Did the slap finally land?

'At the end of my words, I noticed that nothing happened. This person said, "Oh, that's OK. We've got plenty of other people to ask. We just wanted to ask you first."'

'Hey, Yumi, can you volunteer for this thing? It's unpaid, but the exposure will be fantastic for your career!'
'No, thank you. I can't.'

CULTIVATING BIG NO ENERGY

This is some of the shit that Yumi and Claudine's friends have said no to – and survived.

Christmas cards in any form
– PENNY

Ironing or dry cleaning **– CLAIRE**

Making kids go to school on sports days
– VANESSA

The opinions of relatives I don't see or like
– NELLY

People who really aren't interested – it's been quite revolutionary– **VICKI**

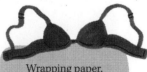

Wrapping paper, cards, wearing a bra
– CARMEL

Wearing a different outfit to the office every day (I have two pairs of black pants in same style and just choose a different top each day) **– FIONA**

Filing my emails!
– TANYA

Pedicures and eyebrow waxing– **EMILY**

Heels – gave them up years ago
– BELINDA

Hair – I shaved my head – **PETA**

Putting deodorant on and brushing my hair – **EVE**

Shaving/waxing legs (unless it's a special occasion) – **SPIKE**

Washing bed sheets every week, most things related to 'housewifery' – **LIBBY**

Baking for any work event – **THEA**

Dusting, ironing, brushing my hair – **NIC**

The dishwasher being packed 'perfectly' – **CAITLIN**

Ironing and anal sex – **ELEESA**

Doing *everything* – **LESLEY**

Feeling the need to fill my weekends with outings and fun activities – **EMMA**

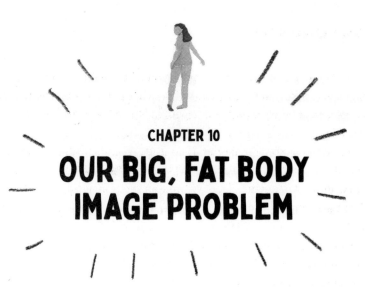

CHAPTER 10

OUR BIG, FAT BODY IMAGE PROBLEM

It doesn't matter if you're fat, thin or in between, the issue of feeling bad about our bodies affects almost all of us.

During high school, writer Bec Shaw would go shopping with her school friends and regularly overhear them in the change room talking about how 'fat and gross' they felt.

'You're in the shop, everyone there knows *I'm* fat and is realising what's happening, but it would never get mentioned,' says Bec. 'Then they would just act as if I was a thin person by complaining about their bodies as though they were scared of being fat, and moaning about how being fat is the worst thing you can be – all while I was there.'

For the duration of the shopping experience, Bec was included as an 'honorary thin person' – presumably so she could be in agreement that being fat was 'the worst!' Bec doesn't think her young friends were trying to be cruel. 'It's so intrinsic and it's so beat into them that it is a moral failing to be fat, and you should feel bad about your body at all times.'

A lot of the discussion around the problem of body image focuses on eating disorders, for good reason. Eating disorders are serious – sometimes deadly – mental illnesses. The Butterfly Foundation reports that **eating disorders affect more than one million Australians, with most cases diagnosed in girls and women.**

What we don't really talk about is garden-variety body DISSATISFACTION, which is a constant mental white noise. Decades of research clearly show that women and girls are more likely to be unhappy about their appearance than feel good about how they look. Most women want to change something about the way they look.

This negative body image affects our self-esteem, makes us act in unhealthy ways, puts us at risk of mental illness and increases our risk of eating disorders. Dissatisfaction with your body doesn't have to develop into something clinical in order to have a profound effect on your life.

Professor Phillippa Diedrichs, a psychologist who uses hard science to champion body positivity and appearance, says we need to take the issue of body image dissatisfaction far more seriously. She goes so far as to call it a public health *emergency*.

Ladies, we need to talk about our BODY IMAGE.

> If you need someone to talk to, call:
>
> **Lifeline** on 13 11 14
> **Butterfly Foundation** on 1800 33 4673
> or visit **National Eating Disorders Collaboration** at nedc.com.au/support-and-services-2/get-help/

✳ ✳ ✳

So, what exactly is 'body image'? It's the relationship you have with your body, and it has four aspects:

What you SEE when you look at yourself (*perceptual* body image). This isn't always accurate!

How you FEEL about your body (*affective* body image). Think of this as a spectrum of satisfaction, which ranges from happiness and enjoyment to disgust and loathing.

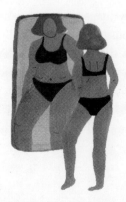

What you THINK about your body (*cognitive* body image). This is where you can start to be preoccupied with the weight and shape of your body.

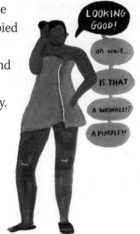

How you BEHAVE because of your body image (*behavioural* body image). If you're dissatisfied with your appearance, you may isolate yourself or engage in unhealthy behaviours to change your appearance.

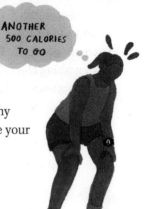

You don't have to love everything about your body all of the time to have positive body image, you just need to be able to *accept* it.

If you look in the mirror, see what is really there and feel mostly OK about it – FANTASTIC! If you can usually appreciate the wonderful things your body does – bloody MARVELLOUS! And if you know, like really *know*, that your worth and value as a human are not determined by how you look – you are RIGHT, and we are fist-pumping and yee-hah-ing for you!

The problem arises when the negative thoughts and feelings about your body outweigh the positive. This is known as body dissatisfaction or negative body image. If this is your experience? We see you.

When making the body image episode of *Ladies, We Need To Talk*, the producers went to the streets to ask women their stories about living with negative body image. It was striking how *real* the real-world consequences were.

Negative body image can inhibit your love life.

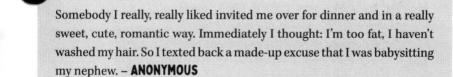

Somebody I really, really liked invited me over for dinner and in a really sweet, cute, romantic way. Immediately I thought: I'm too fat, I haven't washed my hair. So I texted back a made-up excuse that I was babysitting my nephew. – **ANONYMOUS**

Negative body image can stop you from doing what you love.

> I can remember being invited to places like the beach with friends and making up an excuse not to go because I didn't want to be seen in my swimsuit next to those particular friends, who were much thinner and more tanned than I was. I didn't want to be lying on a towel next to them and to have such a direct comparison between my body and theirs. These are some of my closest friends. – **ANONYMOUS**

And negative body image can make you want to hide from yourself.

> As a teenager I would get undressed ... and I'd get in the shower as quickly as possible so that I wouldn't be confronted with myself in the mirror and have to look at my own body because I just hated it so much. – **ANONYMOUS**

Healthy body image matters because it helps you to have good self-esteem and mental health, and helps foster a positive attitude towards eating and physical activity. 'When women and girls feel like they don't look good enough, they are more likely to experience depression, stress and anxiety, engage in unhealthy weight control practices, and exercise too much or too little,' says Professor Diedrichs.

She says body image dissatisfaction is isolating and damages social connections. This isn't just about dating and sexual relationships. Feeling unhappy with your body can also make you keep your distance from family, friends and colleagues. 'We see that with girls not putting their hands up in the classroom. In an extreme case, it is not going to school because they're worried about how they look.'

BODY MASS INDEX

BMI is a calculation used to determine whether you are in a 'healthy weight range' for your height. It is often used with other measurements, such as waist circumference, to figure out if you are at risk of certain illnesses. While it is still used, many argue it isn't an accurate measurement of health and it can be problematic for those at risk of eating disorders.

Then there's the impact on our professional lives. Professor Diedrichs points to two studies in the US and China, each involving thousands of women, which found **women who thought they were overweight (irrespective of what their actual body weight was) were less likely to turn up to job interviews**. They also cited worrying about the way they look as a reason not to go to work. Yumi has a friend who failed hairdressing school because she refused to come out from behind the counter – she was embarrassed about the way her bum looked.

Yet, despite this impact on our lives, those working in the field say that body image is still trivialised. When we struggle with our body image, we're called 'shallow', 'vain' or 'superficial'. We're told to GET OVER IT.

'It's seen as something that's just for silly little girls. What the evidence really suggests is, it's much bigger than that,' says Professor Diedrichs.

DISORDERED EATING

An unhealthy and disturbed eating pattern that can involve dieting, compulsive eating or skipping meals. This can be an indicator of the development of an eating disorder, especially when it involves restrictive dieting.

ORTHOREXIA

Orthorexia is when the idea of 'clean eating' is taken to an extreme. Eating standards become more rigid, tied up with being 'good' or 'bad', to the point of avoiding foods necessary for continued wellbeing.

A BIT MORE ABOUT
EATING DISORDERS

Eating disorders are not a lifestyle choice, an attention-seeking behaviour or a version of 'clean eating'. They are potentially life-threatening mental illnesses, and linked to some very serious medical issues that can affect major organs.

It's helpful to understand that for a lot of people, eating disorders aren't the issue so much as a way of coping with an issue. There are a number of factors that contribute to the development of an eating disorder, including genetics, personality traits, life events or trauma, environment and social factors. Body image dissatisfaction is one factor that can contribute, but you can have an eating disorder and not have poor body image.

Anorexia nervosa is an eating disorder that involves restrictive eating, which can ultimately lead to being unable to maintain a 'normal' and 'healthy' weight, which is determined by your body mass index (BMI). People with anorexia tend to have distorted body image and an intense fear of gaining weight or becoming overweight, regardless of their appearance. Anorexia is the mental illness with the highest mortality rate.

Atypical anorexia has the same diagnostic criteria as anorexia nervosa: restricting kilojoules, intense fear of gaining weight and distorted body image. But unlike anorexia nervosa, those with atypical anorexia have bodies that weigh in within the normal BMI weight range. Over time people with atypical anorexia may become underweight, but even if they don't they are still at risk of malnutrition and health issues.

Body dysmorphic disorder is a mental illness that involves an obsessive focus on perceived flaws in appearance, which causes severe emotional distress. These flaws may be minor, imperceptible to others or non-existent. The person involved will spend considerable amounts of time and/or money trying to fix them. The preoccupation with flaws can be so extreme that the affected person has trouble functioning at work, school or in social situations.

Bulimia nervosa is an eating disorder that involves periods of binge eating followed by some sort of 'compensation' (vomiting, intense exercise or intense dieting). Those with bulimia may also place an excessive emphasis on their body weight or appearance.

Binge eating disorder involves eating large amounts of food over very short periods of time where the person often feels out of control. This can involve eating much more than usual, eating until uncomfortably full or eating large amounts when not hungry. People with binge eating disorder do not engage in 'compensatory' behaviours. More recent research data suggests that binge eating disorder is diagnosed almost as often in males as females.

Other specified feeding or eating disorder (OSFED) involves feeding or eating behaviours that cause distress and have an impact on your life but do not meet the criteria for anorexia, bulimia or binge eating disorder. This is the most common type of eating disorder.

Eating disorders can be difficult to spot because the person with the eating disorder sometimes doesn't know they have one or can be very good at hiding symptoms and evidence. There is a very long list of warning signs of eating disorders, but they broadly fall into three categories.

★ **Physical signs** may include rapid weight loss or change in weight, fainting or dizziness, feeling tired and not sleeping well, or feeling cold even when it is warm.

★ **Psychological signs** may include preoccupation with eating, food, weight or body shape; being anxious or irritable around meal times; feeling out of control around food; or using food as self-punishment.

★ **Behavioural signs** may include dieting, evidence of binge eating, compulsive or excessive exercise, changes in food preference, or secretive behaviour around food.

For more information or if you or anyone you know needs help with an eating disorder, please contact the Butterfly Foundation, Lifeline or visit the National Eating Disorders Collaboration (details on page 146).

Women hating how they look is nothing new. For older women, weight is still the thing they're most unhappy with, but young women now tend to find fault in *every part of themselves.*

Researcher and clinical psychologist Dr Gemma Sharp, who we met way back in the first chapter, says younger women now tend to have a 'global dissatisfaction' when it comes to their appearance. 'I think it's because they believe there are so many things they can change about themselves through cosmetic procedures, which have become more mainstream, whereas in the past, it was more, "Well, I can control my weight, or I can try to, and that will be what I'm dissatisfied with."'

Professor Diedrichs explains how common it is for most women and girls to be dissatisfied with how they look. This widespread body dissatisfaction has a name among researchers: normative discontent.

In research going back to the mid 1980s, Professor Diedrichs says 'we see prevalence rates varying from anywhere between 50 and 90 per cent of women and girls feeling like the way they look is not good enough'.

NORMATIVE DISCONTENT

The notion that the majority of women are unhappy with their appearance, in particular their body weight, and that this is normal.

In the 1990s, the Australian Longitudinal Study on Women's Health found that two-thirds of younger women (between the ages of 18 and 23) whose BMI fell within the range of 'normal' or 'underweight' would still like to lose weight.

Fast-forward to the Mission Australia Youth Survey report in 2020, which found that the top three concerns for young people in Australia were coping with stress, mental health and ... body image. It is staggering to think that body image was still one of the top concerns for young people during a global pandemic where everyone's lives were thrown into chaos and disruption. The survey also showed that body image was more of an issue for young women when compared to young men, with almost half of all young women surveyed saying they were extremely or very concerned about it.

Body image concerns also affect gender diverse people, men and boys, and it appears to be a growing issue. Some experts say we've missed its impact on males because they don't report it and it looks different to how it's experienced by women. But on the whole, body image research is one of the rare medical fields where there's been a greater focus on the female experience. Even those who say we need more research into the male experience admit body image has a profound impact on females.

'For several decades now,' says Professor Diedrichs, 'we've had research showing that girls and women are disproportionately affected by body image concerns, and worrying about the way they look and feeling like they need to look a certain way in order to be successful in life and in society.'

Our body dissatisfaction takes up precious brain space and adds to our mental load.

Professor Diedrichs educated us about BODY CHECKING, a habit many of us have. You probably don't even realise you're doing it. But it's something we tend to do. A lot.

How's my hair?

Is there something in my teeth?

Is my flab showing?

Am I covering my tummy?

BODY CHECKING

Finding ways to quickly check what you look like throughout the day. Also known as 'self surveillance'.

Professor Diedrichs says the idea of body checking stems from 'self-objectification theory'. 'Essentially, as a woman or girl, we start to see ourselves more as objects ... to be looked at by other people, often by men, or through the male gaze. Rather than our bodies being active tools and being really multidimensional.'

Cast your mind back over the last day and think of all the times you've glanced at yourself to get reassurance that you look OK.

This isn't just about looking at yourself in the mirror as you wash your hands. 'It can also be things like when you're sitting at a meeting in the boardroom and you're judging how much space your thighs are taking up in the chair, for example,' says Professor Diedrichs. 'All of these little subtle moments where we're thinking, "OK, how do I look right now? How am I presenting to other people?"'

Body checking steals brain space and energy.

'When it's getting to the point that it's taking up a lot of time, or it's taking your time away from, say, preparing for that meeting, that's when it becomes problematic,' says Professor Diedrichs. 'There's a lot of research showing, as human beings, we're not great at multitasking or moving our attention between different things. If we constantly shift our attention to our appearance, our ability to then engage with the tasks at hand that we're doing may be compromised. It's those incremental moments that count as well.'

The space your thighs take up on a chair, the back fat that might be showing in your dress, the regrowth you glimpsed as you washed your cup in the sink, the nipples showing through your new bra, the fingernails with jagged edges (ugh!) and the zit on your chin that you just spent an hour trying not to stare at on Zoom ... The cumulative impact of that time suck is HUGE.

✳ ✳ ✳

So, when exactly do our body image issues start?

There have been many studies looking at the impact of body image on very young children. A review of 16 studies published in 2016 by Australian researchers found that children as young as six were dissatisfied with their body image. Many of these studies found that it was a greater issue for young girls than younger boys. Professor Diedrichs says research has found that girls as young as three are talking about not wanting to be fat. 'Researchers have found that young schoolgirls tend to be more unhappy with their bodies than boys of the same age, and how young girls feel about their bodies is more likely to have an impact on their mood and self-esteem.'

This rings true for Dr Sneh Tiwari (we met Dr Tiwari in the periods chapter), who was always told she was fat. 'I remember having a nickname in my own language which actually means "fat". On top of this, there were relatives that would comment on my food portions, which made mealtimes uncomfortable.'

Claudine also remembers teasing and comments from her childhood about her weight and how much she was eating. She was a kid who LOVED food, and in hindsight she was using it to self-soothe, but some of the comments people made have stayed with her and to this day she feels a sense of guilt and shame if she eats too much or eats certain foods. She thinks the people who made comments were trying to help her – they wanted her to be happy, and for them that meant being 'slim'.

Then along comes puberty, a time when NO-ONE feels comfortable in their skin. You wake up one morning and *bam!* The Boob Fairy has visited. For some people, this is cool. But ... she brought her goddamn mates: the Zit Fairy, the Period Fairy, the Discharge Fairy, the Hips Fairy, the Thighs Fairy, the B.O. Fairy and, our personal favourite, the Hairy Fairy! (Claudine was also visited by the Bucktooth Fairy. And Yumi was unimpressed to realise that the Boob Fairy somehow skipped her place.)

Both boys and girls start to struggle more with body satisfaction after they hit 11 or 12, but research suggests that by the time they get to 15 or 16, boys tend to develop a bit more self-esteem around their bodies. For girls in their teens, however, body image seems to either plateau or get worse.

Certainly for Dr Tiwari, this was a time when she truly believed she was overweight and unattractive. 'It affected my self-confidence for a long time. Looking back at old pictures from my teenage years with my two adult daughters, they always say I was never overweight or unattractive.'

Unfortunately, body dissatisfaction is not something you just grow out of. Finishing school and going to uni or starting work can be another negative body image trigger – a time when those with mental illness often have their first experience of being unwell. So, too, pregnancy and having kids. But not always.

Claudine hates looking at pictures of herself from her teenage years and still dislikes what she sees. But the turning point in her relationship with her body came in her late 20s when she got pregnant. Once the nausea eased, she noticed that even though pregnancy could be a 'headfuck', her body seemed to know what it had to do. It was like body image rehab.

Yumi's first pregnancy and birth had similar benefits. She'd always felt that being flat-chested was a deficiency and an embarrassment. Then her daughter came and she breastfed, and Yumi looked down at herself and went, 'Fuck it. At least it worked.'

So can we count on body dissatisfaction easing as we age? Nuh-uh. Experts say that for many women, body satisfaction can also take a nosedive in mid-life – at a time when you would hope that you were well and truly comfortable in your own skin. Except that that skin has started to pucker, discolour, sag and grow cancers ... sigh.

There are also plenty of older women who struggle with the impacts of poor body image.

Rosi is 81 years old. She's a woman you'd describe as 'good value' – she's loud, funny and does not give a damn. Still ... 'I was about 12 the first time I wished I was thin. I've practically been on every diet that was ever invented.

'Every time I wanted to get into my bikini I'd go on some crash diet. There was one where you'd have a tin of tomatoes and eat that fried up with a bit of onion and that would be dinner. Every day. I did it for about two weeks. I did the grapefruit diet, and the Atkins, the everything ... My mother and I did a fruit day once a week where you only ate fruit.

'I dieted all my life until I was about 60 and then I thought, "What the hell!"

Despite no longer being on a diet, Rosi's body confidence still isn't great. 'I don't like anything about myself when I look in the mirror. No, seriously. I can't think of anything I like. I hate being fat. I hate having so many wrinkles. I hate my hair thinning.

'I look at young people and think, "If only they realised how lucky they are!"'

When it comes to understanding the factors driving our body image issues, Dr Sharp suggests two theories.

One is known as the tripartite influence model, and yes, it sounds quite academic, but the gist of it is that your family (which includes your parents), your peers and the media are the trio of influences on your body image.

The other is known as self-objectification theory, which Professor Diedrichs mentioned earlier in the chapter. It's not so much about looking in the mirror and thinking 'I look strong' or 'I love this top', but rather 'Do I look sexy?' or 'Would Dev Patel want to bang me?'

Combine the two theories and the influences on our body image include parents, family, peers, past and present partners, society, the patriarchy, the beauty industry (which we'll be focusing on in the next chapter) and the media. That is a *long* list.

While we can't easily control factors like society and the patriarchy, some of these damaging influences are ones we *choose* to consume.

'The media has always had a role to play in how women and people feel about their bodies,' says Dr Sharp. The media is so influential because it reaches so many people and sets a very narrow, and often unattainable, standard of women's physical beauty. When we're served up these body image ideals, we often forget the mainstream media's brutal selection process.

'We tend to be presented with the most beautiful, awesome people in the media. "Regular" people rarely make the cut, so by comparing ourselves to these beautiful and awesome creatures, we compare ourselves to the professionally gorgeous – to those for whom gorgeousness is part of the job description.

'These professionally gorgeous folk are either freakishly good-looking because they have been born like that or because they have significant resources – time and money – to dedicate to the pursuit of gorgeousness.'

Dr Sharp says social media is 'taking this to the next level'. It makes us feel like the awesome and beautiful media people are our peers, which makes it even easier to draw comparisons. Even though every generation faces its challenges, Dr Sharp says things are pretty grim for young people today.

'It does seem to be that we have a youth group coming through who are the most dissatisfied with how they look out of anyone from previous generations. These are the people who have grown up with social media. While we can't say for sure that social media has directly caused this, it does seem to be that we have the most mentally unwell group of young people coming through at the moment.'

Yep, that's pretty grim.

'And now,' she adds, 'we've got all these photo-editing applications.'

This brings us to Snapchat dysmorphia. *CUE DOOM MUSIC* When we talk about young people having it worse than ever, this is the kind of thing we're talking about.

SNAPCHAT DYSMORPHIA

Wanting to look more like your edited, filtered self than your 'real' self.

Snapchat was the first social media platform to introduce in-app photo-editing filters in 2015, and by the following year it had more than 150 million daily users. 'Snapchat dysmorphia' was first identified by a cosmetic doctor in London in 2018.

Dr Sharp thinks it could as easily be called 'Instagram dysmorphia'. 'We found that 97 per cent of young girls were on Instagram, and Instagram has the same filters now … **About 40 per cent were almost always filtering their photos before they posted them.** So about two in five were like, "There's no way I'd put up an unfiltered photo of myself. Ever."

To the list you can now add Zoom dysmorphia, with many of us spending hours each day using video conferencing tools and applying filters to improve our appearance.

'They go to cosmetic surgeons and ask to look like their filtered photo. The cosmetic surgeon has to say, "I can't actually make you look like that. That's a photo-editing application. It's thinned down your nose, it's cleared and brightened your skin and widened your eyes."

'Before people would take in pictures of celebrities saying, "Make me look like Kim Kardashian," but now they're taking in pictures of *themselves.*'

There are even apps that simulate plastic surgery procedures on your photos. The problem is that even though these changes are easy to make within a photo-editing app, it's a very different story on an actual human body using surgery. Plastic surgeons themselves caution against the use of cosmetic surgery apps, especially among younger people, because they downplay the risks, pain and costs of surgery, and also fuel appearance pressures.

Despite all the damage it is doing to our body image, Dr Sharp still believes there are ways to use social media as a 'tool for good'. She's looking to see if mindfulness principles, such as pausing and holding a non-judgemental perspective, can help. And working with a team at the Butterfly Foundation, she's helped to develop KIT, the world's first positive body image chatbot.

'What I and other researchers are trying to do is teach people to be mindful when they use social media and teach them to be more critical of what they're seeing. To take a step back from what they're viewing and asking, "Is this actually helpful? Is this even a real picture?"

'It's about teaching people higher levels of thought when engaging with social media instead of just consuming it in the passive way that we often do.'

Dr Sharp and the Butterfly Foundation have some suggestions for how to navigate social media in a positive way:

* Make connections, not comparisons.
* Follow a diverse range of people and accounts.
* Pay attention to how you feel after you use social media.
* Limit your time on social media when you're feeling down.

Instagram gets a really bad rap but one thing that has really, really helped me is body-positive accounts on Instagram. Seeing bigger-bummed girls just wearing whatever they want, looking sexy and confident – it really has helped me.

Seeing women embrace their curves and their rolls and their cellulite has changed my life. Like, it has got into my subconscious almost. I am more than just my flabby stomach. It really doesn't matter. What I look like doesn't determine how valuable I am or how intelligent I am and I can contribute so much more to society and have more fun in life if I'm not just focusing on my body. – **ANONYMOUS**

✳ ✳ ✳

Being more mindful of how you use social media is one of the ways you can help create a better body image culture for yourself. But you also need to take that mindfulness and compassion beyond social media platforms.

While it's highly unlikely that you say cruel things to people about their appearance, there's a good chance you make terrible comments about yourself – things like 'my hair is gross' or 'I can't stand my fat arms'. If you are saying mean things about your body out loud then pretty soon someone nearby will hear and internalise your words.

Bec Shaw's experiences of girls trashing their own bodies in her friendship group didn't end in high school. She still notices that once someone starts talking among friends about how they feel about their body, someone else will chime in and then another person. 'I think it's so contagious because it's a quick way to bond with another woman,' she says. 'We don't encourage women and young women to celebrate the way they look – so what they are also doing is sending out signals, "I don't like my body. It's OK, don't tease me. Don't take me down. I hate myself."

'There's this comedy sketch of women in a circle all taking turns to say something bad about themselves – and it's just escalating and escalating until one of their heads explodes off! It's like you have to say something bad about yourself to be in this group!'

What Bec is describing is known as 'fat talk', and it used to make fat activist Ally Garrett angry. These days she tries to have empathy.

'You're having a bad day, your self-esteem is not good today, or you feel uncomfortable in your body? That's fine,' says Ally. 'But by complaining about having a "fat day"? "Oooh, I'm so fat today!"? The way you're describing it is that *your body looks more like mine today.* For a while that would make me really angry, it would feel like a betrayal and I'd want to leave that conversation.

'But lately, I really have been working on having empathy in those moments, because we're all in this

FAT TALK

The constant negative remarks that people make about fat, body shape and weight, whether their own or others'.

THIN PRIVILEGE

The privilege given to people who are thin and conform to appearance ideals. It mean they can go about their lives knowing they fit in. They can find clothes their size on the racks of clothing shops. People won't shame them for eating a piece of cake in public. Their doctor won't treat every appointment as a weight-loss coaching session.

together. We all live in the same society that feeds us these messages about fat bodies. I'm trying to have empathy that that person is feeling bad about themselves. But I do wish that people wouldn't use the word "fat" to say they feel like shit.'

Research has found that fat talk is contagious and harmful – and not just to those who might be listening in. A 2011 US study entitled 'If You're Fat, Then I'm Humongous!' found that college women who engaged in fat talk were likely to experience higher levels of body dissatisfaction and guilt than those who didn't.

It's well past time to stop fat talk; let's start talking positively about our bodies and focus a LOT less on how they look. Dr Sharp suggests we talk to ourselves like we would a friend: with *compassion*. 'Because you would never say anywhere near the stuff to them that you would say to yourself.'

Dr Sharp is a fan of affirmations. Here are a few to take with you.

- ★ **My weight is not my worth.** 'It's really important to remember that a number on the scale is not who you are,' says Dr Sharp. 'It literally is a number on the scale. It's about detaching from that number and not giving it the airtime anymore.'
- ★ **Function over form.** Remember to appreciate the amazing things your body does for you (breathe, exercise, have sex) and not just focus on the shell it comes in. Being a great dancer, hugger, lover or fighter has nothing to do with being fat, thin, big-bosomed, tanned or free of cellulite.
- ★ **I am more than my body.** I am a person who ran a half-marathon! I am a person who organised that food drive. I am a sexy horndog. I am a daughter who has a functional and loving relationship with her parent. I am a funny bitch. I am a great friend.

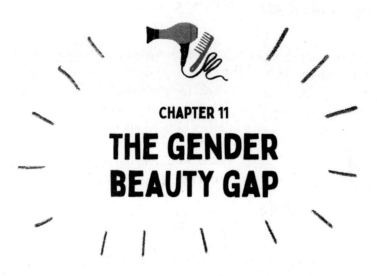

CHAPTER 11

THE GENDER BEAUTY GAP

his is a boring trope and we've seen it a million times, but we're going to describe it anyway.

There's a guy waiting for a girl. She's taking ages to get ready. He's downstairs, neat and shiny and radiant with anticipation. His hair is combed. He waits. The clock ticks. What is she DOING up there?

His eyes dart around. There is nothing he can do to be more ready. He waits.

Finally! She appears, stepping down carefully in a waft of chiffon and hairspray. He gasps. The wait was ... worth it! She is MAGNIFICENT.

It's no secret that women spend more time and money on the way we look than men. But have we ever added it all up? Like, seriously, sat down and tallied up the hours and dollars?

Because you know how some women hide make-up receipts from their partners? (It sounds cheesy and archaic, but it happens.) Well, some of us hide the grooming receipts – from *ourselves*.

We accept that the effort that goes into looking magnificent – or, at the very least, 'put together' – is one of the many costs of being a woman. But we rarely confront head-on the sum total of these costs.

From when we're young, it's expected that we will use a range of products and treatments to be as beautiful as we can be. It's assumed we're willing to spend big on make-up, skincare and serums, haircuts and colours, blow waves and styling, facials, Botox and fillers, teeth whitening, eyebrow treatments and eyelash extensions, hair removal, manicures and pedicures ... And at the risk of stating the painfully obvious, this expectation does not extend to men.

It's not just money – although it costs us a good chunk of our earnings.

It's not just time – although we lose too much of this precious resource to it.

It's time AND money, plus *mental energy*. The same mental energy that we've already overdrawn.

Ladies, have you noticed that we are being royally screwed by the GENDER BEAUTY GAP?

Let's start with money. The beauty industry is serious big bucks. It's hard to know exactly how much we're spending, but a few market research surveys give us a clue. For instance, in 2014 an Ipsos survey of 1001 women in Australia found they spent close to $3600 a year on beauty products, on average. (This same survey found four out of five women hide their beauty purchases from their partners or loved ones.)

Then in 2016 a survey by an Australian financial comparison website found that **Australian women spend $15 billion annually on products and services that improve appearance,** including beauty products, make-up, professional hair colouring, and skincare products and treatments. During the same period men spent $2.08 billion on grooming costs, such as shaving and beard trimming.

These figures didn't include fashion, cosmetic surgery, wellness, fitness or other types of self-care that can improve appearance. Of course there are women who choose not to spend money on beauty and appearance, but there are also those who spend far more than $3600 a year. Much, much more.

Let's look beyond the money. There is also the time and mental energy that goes into our appearance. The time spent planning and organising grooming appointments. Time spent shopping for affordable beauty products that work. The amount of trial and error that goes into getting the colour of your foundation right. The brain space it takes to figure out how the hell you fit all of this in with all the other important things you need to do.

This is harder to quantify, and there doesn't seem to be any data to help us understand these costs. So we're going to take a look at the lives of a few different women to get a better sense of what the gender beauty gap actually looks like.

A SHORT SURVEY ON THE COST OF BEAUTY

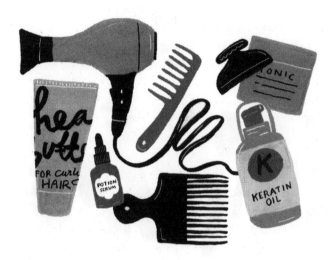

Sarah works in the public service and says she's quite into beauty: make-up, serums and creams, treatments and fillers.

Her big thing is her hair. 'My hair has always been extremely curly and thick. My mom is half African American, half Belgian, and my dad is white. I was born with basically a big, curly afro and since 12 or 13 I've had straightening treatments. I've been having them more regularly in the last 10 years.'

★ **Time:** At least an hour each morning on her hair and make-up (which, over the course of a year, adds up to about 45 eight-hour workdays). Sarah doesn't resent this time; in fact, she sees this as 'me time' – the only part of the day that she gets to herself, while her husband looks after their young daughters. Then there's the time she spends washing and styling her hair (a couple of times a week), doing hair treatments at home (every month or so) and heading to the hairdresser. Sarah also has other semi-regular beauty appointments (injectables, laser hair removal, etc.).

* **Money:** Sarah estimates that she spends about $6000 a year on products and treatments. By far the biggest portion of her grooming spend is for her hair. None of this includes the money she spends on clothes and fashion, her other loves.
* **Mental energy:** Sarah has mixed feelings about her beauty regimen. On the one hand, it's her opportunity to put her needs first, but on the other, she is aware of the example it sets for her daughters and admits that it does take up quite a bit of her headspace.
* **What she'd love to stop doing:** None of it. If money was no object, she reckons she'd get a personal hairstylist – like the Kardashians.

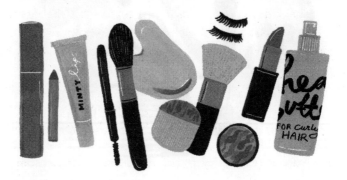

Emma Husar was a federal MP between 2016 and 2019. During her time in parliament she found herself scrutinised in ways she never anticipated. Even though no-one told her she had to look a certain way, she felt pressure to 'conform and to throw on a face full of make-up'. If she didn't, she knew it would be one more thing people could comment on and criticise.

But Emma was ALSO told (by a former senior politician) not to look 'too pretty' – 'because female voters would be threatened and insecure if their husbands wanted to vote for me.'

* **Time:** Emma had to spend a lot of time maintaining the highly professional polished appearance that matched her electoral posters. (True story: it's expected that politicians will look like the pictures on their posters for years after the photo was taken.) Getting ready for public appearances took hours. Emma remembers being in the make-up chair before a regular TV appearance and seeing a male colleague arrive to do an earlier segment. 'He had come in, done his hair and

make-up, which was literally powder on his nose for maybe 10 seconds, done his interview, come back and said goodbye and left. I hadn't even got out of the make-up chair yet.'

★ **Money:** 'Before going into politics, I hardly wore any make-up. My sister used to order my make-up for me, and about halfway through my term she said, "What are you doing with this stuff? Eating it?" Because suddenly I was using so much more makeup than I ever had before. I hadn't even realised. It had become such a part of my routine that I was just putting it on every day.'

★ **Mental energy:** Expectations she faced around her appearance made it impossible to just 'pop into the shops to buy milk or bread', so Emma enlisted her kids to run errands for her as she sat in the car outside. It took energy, effort and brain space to come up with this solution. Not to mention the effort required to convince teenagers to walk into the shop and buy milk and bread!

★ **What she'd love to stop doing:** Like Sarah, Emma has curly hair and spends hours blow-drying and styling it. When she was in public life, this was a daily job. 'You have to decide "Am I going to exercise today or am I going to blow-dry my hair?" Because I can't exercise then run under a shower (like the men can) and go down to the chamber.'

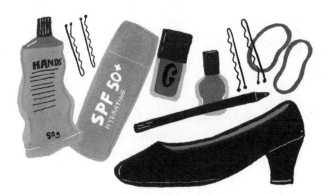

Olivia works in an industry notorious for its beauty standards. As an air hostie, the beauty 'rules' are official and almost punitive.

For instance, Olivia and her female colleagues can have short hair and wear it out until it touches their shoulders. At this point, it must be tied up in a ponytail *but* the hair elastic must be covered AT ALL TIMES, either by hair wrapped around it or a ponytail shield. Once a ponytail is more than 30 centimetres long, it must be tied up into a neat twisted bun. Nail polish is compulsory (in a range of four colours that match the uniform) and it can't be chipped.

'I just wish people would understand that the reason I am there is because of a legal requirement and that is to evacuate all passengers within 90 seconds,' says Olivia.

Although we're talking about beauty products, it's worth mentioning that Olivia must wear unladdered hosiery and shoes with a heel between 3 and 10 centimetres whenever she is in uniform – even if she has finished her shift and has to walk a few kilometres from the aircraft to her parked car.

- ★ **Time:** Hard to tally up, to be honest. A full face of make-up (foundation, blush, eye shadow, mascara and lipstick or lip gloss) needs to be applied before going to work and then reapplied during the flight. 'Touch up before touchdown' is a saying Olivia was taught during her training – even though their focus is supposed to be looking after the safety and wellbeing of passengers at 10,000 feet.
- ★ **Money:** Olivia's back-of-an-envelope calculation for how much she spends to conform to these standards is about $1500 a year. She gets no allowance and none of these items are tax deductible ... unless they are 'hydrating'.
- ★ **Mental energy:** For Olivia, it's not just the mental energy that's required before and during the flight to ensure she's looking 'perfect' at all times, it's also thinking ahead to make sure her nails, hair and make-up are ready before she starts her shift.
- ★ **What she'd love to stop doing:** If Olivia were writing new standards, she'd immediately make nail polish and make-up optional. (She'd also ditch the archaic rules about heels.) Then she'd use the time she saved to get more sleep, especially on those mornings when she has to get up at 3 am. 'I feel frustrated in this industry that my male colleagues are getting more sleep than I am. They're not spending as much money as I am and I'm just spending more time dealing with that kind of stuff than my male colleagues are.'

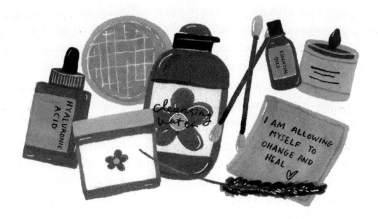

Allira Potter is a Yorta Yorta model, writer, reiki practitioner and mindset coach, who's had to 'unlearn' what she thinks about herself and her body, especially after her intense experiences of bullying in high school. 'If I'm preaching confidence, then it'll help the next female beside me embrace who they are and what they have.'

She'd never really given much thought to the gender beauty gap until she asked herself why she was spending so much time on her appearance. For her the answer 'came down to social media and keeping up with "social norms"'.

* **Time**: At least 20 minutes every night. 'My skin specialist is always drilling me about cleansing and scrubbing at night-time, so once a day is absolutely enough.' But Allira's beauty routine is about more than what she puts on her skin. 'It keeps me in check because I look after my body from the inside out. I know that having a beauty routine is only going to help amplify everything.'
* **Money**: A few hundred dollars per month. 'I don't spend a lot on beauty because I only need a few intense products to help with my skin and body.'
* **Mental energy**: For Allira, time spent on this routine is very much about being mindful about looking after herself.
* **What she'd love to stop doing**: Not much at all because it's all self-care. 'I love my beauty routines, it's important for me to take time out to do this for myself.'

Even for those lucky enough to not have rules – official or unspoken – around how we're expected to groom for our work, we still do it. Why? Well … the patriarchy. It's been hardwired into us that this is what is *expected* of women.

Be it at work, in our relationships or moving through the world, Professor Phillippa Diedrichs (who we met in the previous chapter) says the stakes are high for women when it comes to beauty. 'For girls and women still today, their appearance is used as a way for them to demonstrate their worth and their success,' she says.

'Men can gain what we call "masculine capital", or value, or credit or protection in other ways. That might be through their knowledge, their attributes, through other skills. They can compensate if they don't meet society's standards for what's good-looking.'

Professor Diedrichs says 'for women, it's fundamental that you look a certain way to be considered beautiful or attractive or successful. Women are heavily penalised if we don't meet that standard.'

Our appearance isn't just a measure of our attractiveness. It's seen to be a measure of a range of unrelated qualities, like how motivated we are, how proactive we are, or how much willpower we have.

As Emma Husar says, 'This all comes down to how society thinks about, speaks about and respects women.'

Then there are also the cases where caring TOO MUCH about your appearance leaves women open to criticism. One of the few workplaces in the world where women wearing little or no make-up is standard, is in academia. A little is OK, but too much is considered 'frivolous'.

It's another situation where women can't win.

I wanted to share my own story of the gender beauty gap but where someone felt the need to comment on the fact that I *was* wearing make-up!

It was during my PhD at a medical research institute in Melbourne. I had a late night the evening before and so I was coming into work 'late' (10 am!) and I encountered one of my male colleagues. We made small talk where I felt the need to point out that I knew I was 'late', because I'm a woman and I've been conditioned to always assume everyone is judging me and try to pre-empt it. His response was, 'Oh you can't be running too late because you had time to put on make-up.'

I was just so shocked by this statement that I didn't even respond. I had put a swipe of eyeliner on and that was it and yet he still felt like he had a right to comment on my appearance. And this isn't an uncommon judgement in the world of academia where you [read: female] can be judged for putting too much effort into your appearance because that translates to you not working hard enough on your research. Of course this standard never applies to men.

I just thought by sharing this I could point out that the bar is constantly shifting for women. 'Beauty' is a constantly moving target and it feels like we're damned if we do and damned if we don't. – **CASEY**

Professor Diedrichs is often asked: 'Why is it such a bad thing that I spend time and money on my appearance or on beauty, particularly if it makes me feel good about the way that I look? What's so wrong with that?'

'It may be that we do find it fun to get dressed up and to wear make-up and use our appearance as a source of play, but then [we need to] think critically if it's taking a lot of time and diverting our attention or our money away from other things that we value more in life.'

There's nothing wrong with expressing your identity through the clothes you wear, make-up, hairstyle or other types of adornment on the body like tattoos or piercings. You may choose to wear green eyeliner (like Yumi) or get foils in your hair (like Claudine) because you like the way they look and they make you feel good.

But Professor Diedrichs says there are questions worth asking yourself:

- ★ Why do you feel the need to do these things?
- ★ Why does it make you feel better?
- ★ If you think about it as a type of armour or protection, why is that?

If it turns out that your motivation is to 'not stand out', to 'fit in' or to defend yourself against judgement, then you need to ask yourself if you want to keep doing it.

Sarah (who tallied up her beauty cost for us on page 163) tried to shrink the gender beauty gap in her life. As an experiment, we asked her to ditch all her beauty routines, including basic make-up and hair styling, for just two weeks. Sarah says it was only possible because she was on maternity leave, but even with a baby and toddler, the time she saved not doing her normal grooming meant that she had time to start meditating.

'I've actually come to appreciate natural beauty a lot more. I think that it's been a really positive thing. It's nice to look in the mirror, and be like, "Wow, I can actually feel really positive about my natural beauty."

'Before, I would have thought, "I'm just going out without make-up, ugh!" But now I'm thinking, "Oh, wow, I don't look so bad."'

I am in construction and did a construction degree (not just a sales girl, as many initially think). I am confident to say I am extremely competent at my job but I only wear make-up when meeting clients. My mum never wore make-up, except lipstick when she went out, so I was never obsessed with it. Growing up I never felt make-up did enough for me to make it worth the amount of time it took to put on. I would never look like an Insta model so I thought, 'Why waste the time?'

Working in a largely male-dominated industry, I have felt really strongly that my ability should prove that I am good enough to be in the room, rather than my appearance, and in a way it's pushed me further away from wearing make-up. I believe my mum's relationship with make-up has been the driving factor to how I see myself. I am concerned for my niece who cares so much about her appearance and she is only nine. – (ANOTHER) **SARAH**

While COVID had plenty of downsides for women, one upside was that it changed how many of us approached our beauty routines.

For Claudine, COVID seems to have permanently changed the shape of her days. She's still got a day job, and for that she's grateful, but for most of 2020 she was part of the ABC's team covering COVID and working from her bedroom or her kitchen table.

Initially it felt liberating to wear slippers all day and not have to worry about how she looked, but as the months dragged on, it felt pretty bloody miserable and fairly grey and boring (much like her hair after six months of no visits to the hairdresser).

She's learnt that wearing a cool shirt, a bit of mascara and lip gloss on workdays, even when she doesn't leave the house, helps her to separate her work from non-work life. It's given her a sense that mentally she is still getting out there even if it is only via Zoom.

Lockdown showed Yumi that when she was just with her immediate family, she didn't engage with a lot of the adornment and body decorating that she had previously believed she found 'fun'.

It led her to think: 'If I really believed it was such a terrific form of self-expression, why didn't I do any of it when I didn't have to? Did my need to "express" dissipate with my need to leave the house? Or did my need to conform to beauty standards dissipate when I no longer had to front up in person?'

She's realised that in a work context, she doesn't particularly want to engage with being 'beautiful' or 'plain'. She wants to be known for the work she does. If she wants to go full vamp hoe for a party, that's her business! The hope is that her current beauty regimen – where it's not much but not nothing – attracts the least amount of attention, allowing her work to speak for itself. Much like it would for a man.

This is called 'body neutrality', and it's based on the idea that the way we look is the least interesting and least important thing about us.

Body neutrality doesn't cheerlead appearance positivity, like 'I love my stretch marks! I love my wrinkles! I love my spare tyres!' It doesn't try to translate every detail of our appearance into prettiness or a 'yay!' party. But our bodies are worthy of respect regardless of whether they fit the mould of current beauty ideals.

If COVID didn't force you into a beauty gap circuit-breaker, it's not too late to try an experiment like Sarah's. Take a short break from your usual beauty routine for a few weeks and pay attention to how it makes you feel. It will give you a chance to figure out what makes you feel good and what you do as habit.

This issue has been bothering me my entire adult life, but I never had the vocabulary to talk about it. Thanks for giving me that.

These strange COVID times have had a silver lining for me. In the fear and panic of the first few weeks of lockdown I had a YOLO moment and shaved my head. I have always wanted to, but was too afraid of what people would think. Eight weeks later I'm halfway to a pixie cut and am so happy with my decision. For the first time in my life I don't need to worry about getting my hair wet. I can't style it anyway! This little insight into a man's life has made me start to think about other 'man shortcuts'. I'll report back if I find any.

At the end of the episode you asked what we can do about this. I don't have the answer, but my one suggestion is to change the adjectives we use to describe women.

All the time I hear my wonderful female friends and colleagues described firstly as 'beautiful' ... they are so much more than that. The first word used to describe a man is almost never handsome. You would start with 'smart', 'funny', 'quiet', 'cheeky', etc. I'm hoping that if we shift the focus away from a woman's appearance, there will be more room to see their other attributes and hopefully diversify their social capital.
– RACHEL

✳ ✳ ✳

We're not just talking about mascara here. The gender beauty gap is only one of the many gender gaps that hold women back. There's the gender pay gap, the superannuation gap, the orgasm gap (more on that very soon), the gender leadership gap, the research gap, the fitness gap ... we could go on.

These are examples of the economic, social and political structures that work against gender equality – and that we can fight to change. The choices we make will impact those who follow.

It's worth reminding ourselves that while all women and non-binary people experience discrimination, injustices are served in different-sized portions, depending on who you are.

When Allira Potter was growing up, there was a profound lack of Indigenous representation in the beauty industry and magazines. 'There were no Aboriginal women in that space. We were always in the sports space and thought of as strong, athletic women like Cathy [Freeman]. There wasn't any diversity in the [beauty] industry.'

Allira decided to change that. 'I saw a gap and thought, "I'm pretty like these size 6 blondes, I'm attractive and I can do what they're doing." I came into the modelling industry being like, "I'm doing this for me but I'm also doing this for all the other women too."'

'I do believe the media in general plays a huge part in this because we never really see ads about men's products and how they can take care of themselves.'

And she's not size 6 nor is she turning herself inside out to fit into the world of white modelling. Allira is black and sexy and proud.

Is changing from within, like Allira has done, the answer? How can we all be more like her and not just accept the 'ideals' that we see held up around us but be active agents for change? What does change *look* like when it comes to the gender beauty gap?

Emma Husar thinks change would ideally look like 'awesome, super-confident women who believe, "I'm going to own this and this is me and take it or leave it. This is what I'm comfortable doing. I don't feel any additional pressure." But that takes massive amounts of self-esteem and self-confidence.

'I think, most importantly, [we need] other women in the sisterhood going "good on you", clapping for you, because that is an awesome thing to do.'

This clearly can't just be about individuals – it needs to be about making change TOGETHER.

'I think that when we talk about gender equality, we often look at the men,' says Emma. 'But in my experience, it's sometimes the sisterhood that's not always the most supportive of each other. To our detriment, because the patriarchy rewards whoever plays in it.'

So back your sisters. There's already enough pulling us down. Resist the urge to criticise, especially based on appearance. Much like the 'fat talk' we discussed in the body image chapter, we need to be conscious of the things we say – about others and about ourselves. Not only can our words unintentionally upset people, but they also help to reinforce a culture where it's OK to judge people based on how they look.

Stop using words like 'gorgeous' and 'beautiful' to describe people as though that's the thing that matters most. Especially around little girls, who may be better served hearing words like 'smart', 'fierce', 'natural leader', 'scary' and 'witchy-poo'!

If you don't like what a brand or an organisation is doing by objectifying a female body, mocking appearance or belittling women, tell them. If you don't like a company's advertising or their policies, don't consume their products. Talk about your actions with others. Be like the schoolyard gossip, but angrier.

INTERNALISED MISOGYNY

When women being degraded is so normalised that women internalise it, subconsciously projecting sexist ideas onto other women and even onto themselves.

Professor Diedrichs believes we need to exercise power as consumers to push for change. 'We have a tool for activism in our back pockets with our smartphones ... You can communicate directly with brands and call them out when you think they're doing something that is harmful. Or you can praise them when you think they're doing something well.'

Yumi's advice is to send that email. She's seen multiple examples of bosses in the corporate world treating written correspondence like a big deal – they assume that for every email complaint they receive, there are a hundred people equally pissed off who never got around to writing one. So your email is worth a hundred.

While you're at it, write to your elected representatives and get them to do their bit. Do we need gender quotas in your preferred political party that will help with unfair image expectations on female politicians? What about legislation that will strangle rules about uniform and dress codes that unfairly punish women? Push your representative. They are meant to represent you. You're allowed to be annoying.

We're fully aware that we're talking not to those who created the problem here, but to the very people who are living with the impact of it. This is a huge endeavour to take on, and for some of us it will feel like yet another bloody job to do. Is it time for a revolution? Claudine and Yumi say yes! But actually, we are both very busy – can we schedule in the revolution for next month?

Maybe a good place to start – right now – is by reflecting on the standards we set for ourselves. Look at yourself in the mirror and relax. You don't have to be hot or sexy or a babe. You just have to be you.

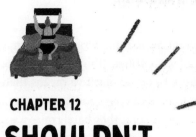

CHAPTER 12

SEX SHOULDN'T HURT - EVER

S *omething was just rawly rubbing inside of me.*

Most times I have sex, it creates some level of pain.

It was all about him thinking he needed to go very, very, very far.

Just a burning pain, it was unbearable.

Like sandpaper, extremely painful pressure, tearing, a horrible and scary experience.

There have been so many times where I've gone, 'This is actually hurting and I need it to stop', so I have faked an orgasm to get them to go.

Stories of painful sexual intercourse are some of the toughest to share. And even when women are talking about something completely unrelated, there's often a serve of painful sex on the side.

Before we go any further, let's be super clear on one thing. Sex should never hurt.

It's important to truly understand this, so we're going to say it again: sex should NEVER hurt.

It's true. Fair dinkum. No joke. Sex should NOT cause you pain. Not even a *little* bit. (OK, there is one caveat: you might enthusiastically consent to certain activities during sex that cause you pain. If that's your jam, cool. That is the ONLY time sex has to hurt.)

The problem is, too many of us have picked up the message that it's completely normal and, in fact, bog-standard to put up with pain during sexual intercourse.

Lili Loofbourow is a staff writer at *Slate* magazine who wrote a viral article about painful sex, entitled 'The female price of male pleasure'. She points out that our desire to be sex-positive means there is a tendency for us to shout from the rooftops about our good sexual experiences. But the bad experiences? Well, for a lot of reasons, they barely raise a whisper.

'Painful sex is a lot more common than I think anyone realises. Again, it's not often discussed because it's kind of shameful. People feel like there's something wrong with them,' says Loofbourow.

What? Another thing women are just meant to silently endure?

Ladies, we need to talk about PAINFUL SEX.

✳ ✳ ✳

If we're going to have a conversation about painful vaginal intercourse, then it's useful to know the medical term for it: *dyspareunia*. For many women, this pain is short-lived and happens rarely, but for others, pain with sex is more … routine.

It's difficult to know exactly how common dyspareunia is. In the most recent Australian Study of Health and Relationships, based on data collected in 2013, researchers found that **17 per cent of women, compared to 1.5 per cent of men, had experienced painful sex for at least one month in the last year.** The American College of Obstetricians and Gynecologists look at it in a slightly different way, saying that 75 per cent of women experience painful sex at some point during their lives.

Loofbourow is confident we don't have an accurate picture of how common painful sex is. 'On PubMed, there are almost four times as many clinical trials on male sexual pleasure as there are on female sexual pain.' Specifically, there were 393 clinical trials studying dyspareunia, 10 on vaginismus and 43 on vulvodynia (more about these conditions very soon). For erectile dysfunction there were 1954. While there has been an increase in clinical trials in the last few years, the stats are very clear.

We don't want to go too far down this rabbit hole, but this lack of interest in women's health issues is everywhere in medical research. It's known as (drum roll …) the research gap. For many years, all research opportunities and funding went to straight white males. They were the ones deciding on the issues worthy of being interrogated. So if you are not a member of this club – that is, if you are female or gender diverse, not white, not hetero –

well, there are a bunch of things about your experience that we just don't have the answers for. The next time someone tries to (man)splain to you that something you are experiencing isn't real because there is no evidence that it exists, ask them if there has been any research on the subject or whether no-one has bothered to even ask the questions.

'The medical community spends a lot of energy making sure that men who can't get erections are able to somehow achieve them. But it's *not* especially worried about women having extreme pain when they're having intercourse,' says Loofbourow. 'There are reasons for that having to do with the pharmaceutical industry – where research dollars come from and where they go. But god, I think people are really underestimating the number of women who would invest in products that would help them have less painful sex.'

When men and women talk about bad sex, they're talking about wildly different things, according to Loofbourow. 'Bad sex for men tends to mean that they didn't have an orgasm, or they were bored. For women, bad sex often means tearing or pain, or any number of emotionally violating experiences.'

The expectation that women should be willing to suffer through penetrative sex with gritted teeth is set up from the very first time we do it. It's not just accepted, it's completely *normalised* that our first time will be painful.

It doesn't have to be this way.

Dr Anita Elias is Head of the Sexual Medicine and Therapy Clinic in Melbourne, and has been seeing women who experience painful sex for more than 20 years. 'Sex should never be painful. If you're having painful sex, there's something going on that needs to be sorted out,' she says.

Because sex involves the BODY and the BRAIN, Dr Elias says painful sex is often a mix of physical *and* psychological factors. 'How you feel, what you're thinking, affects what's happening physically in the body. And the other way around. If sex hurts, why would you want to do it? So what's happening physically is affecting how you feel and how you think – you really can't separate them.'

We know there are plenty of ways sex can be awful that have nothing to do with pain. Loofbourow says she wants to focus on the physical aspects of the pain, because while we're slowly opening up the conversation about the emotional aspects of sexual encounters, we're still NOT talking about the fact that women tear, bleed or feel like they are being stabbed in the bowel during sex. 'If you're bleeding after an experience that's supposed to be pleasurable, this seems like something we should be talking about.'

* * *

The most common cause of painful sex is sadly unremarkable. It's not a gigantic mystery. It's not an incurable medical issue.

'The most common thing I see is not being turned on enough, leading to dryness in the vagina,' says Dr Elias.

One of the things Claudine and Yumi discussed on that first coffee date was the fact that NOBODY TALKS ABOUT what happens to women's bodies when they become sexually aroused. It's pretty much something you have to figure out for yourself as you go along. But if your early experiences of sex are dry and painful, how and when do you learn this vitally important lesson?

For a woman to enjoy vaginal intercourse (regardless of how many times she has done it and regardless of what is being inserted in her vagina), she needs to be aroused and lubricated. Physical signs of arousal for women include an increased heart rate, the nipples hardening, the vulva and vagina filling with blood and becoming puffy and engorged ... and the vagina becoming lubricated or wet.

When you're aroused, your vagina and the glands around the vaginal entrance – the Bartholin's and Skene's glands – secrete fluids that reduce friction and create a lovely slippery sensation that allows for penetration without pain.

If you're NOT sufficiently aroused before penetration, your vagina will probably feel dry and you may experience a feeling of friction, burning, stinging, tearing or throbbing.

I had no idea that discharge actually has a purpose – sexual lubrication! I didn't even know this the first time I had sex. I had no idea there was ANY preparation on the woman's side in terms of getting lubricated. In fact, I was actually cleaning away any discharge before penetration because I thought my boyfriend would be grossed out. I literally just thought you stuck the penis in and then got magical orgasms. You can imagine my disappointment when it was just a sore, painful experience! – **RACHEL**

There are plenty of things that can affect arousal, but often it's about lack of foreplay and the associated failure to allow enough time for the vagina to become lubricated.

It's an issue that comes up for couples of all ages and stages. It's all too common to rush to penetration before the woman is ready, particularly in younger, more inexperienced couples. It's also a pretty big issue in hook-up sex, when there often isn't much rapport between the two players. They don't know your body and you don't know theirs. Communication is key for this type of sex to be great – but that can feel like a large investment for a small return.

At the other end of the relationship spectrum, lubrication can be an issue for long-term committed and loving couples. Sometimes it's about complex relationship problems or mismatched libido. But it can also be some tiny detail, like that as foreplay starts, you realise you can smell their bum because they haven't wiped properly. In that case? Yeah, it's going to be hard to get turned on. (This has happened.)

At certain times in your cycle or during certain life stages, such as after birth or while breastfeeding, hormonal changes can also make it harder to get wet when you're horny. One of the key symptoms of menopause – a dry vagina – can make for very painful sex. It's from falling oestrogen levels, which make the skin of your vagina thinner, less elastic and less moist. As intercourse starts to become painful, you can become quite anxious about sex and this can set up a negative 'pain cycle'.

None of these problems are impossible to overcome – knowing your body and understanding how it works will empower you to find the answers you need. But you might need to see a doctor to figure out the best solution for you.

I haven't menstruated now for six years and had a pretty cruisy menopause overall. I still get hot flushes, but other than that, life has gone on much the same as ever. Oh, except for my dry vagina!

I have been in a very happy marriage for 36 years, and my husband and I have together enjoyed a great sex life. So to suddenly have painful sex was not something either of us were enjoying. For me it was obviously painful, for my husband he was terrified of hurting me. Lube made no difference. Foreplay and using a vibrator to get things 'moist and opened up' helped a bit. I tried a pessary with some success. I tried oestrogen cream with similar success. For five-and-a-half years we battled with this problem, feeling frustrated and upset. We both still wanted to have comfortable, spontaneous sex, and missed it.

What I didn't understand, although I probably should have, considering I am a nurse, is that it isn't just a matter of dryness, but of the thinning of the walls of the vagina. You can use a whole tube of lube – it won't make a bit of difference to changing these ageing, thinning vagina walls. Your podcast episode thankfully touched on this issue. Talking with colleagues at work who have gone through menopause, this appears to be a very common problem, with a number of women giving up sex completely because of the discomfort or pain.

A few months ago, during a visit to my doctor, she told me she had recently been to a conference on this very issue. The 'latest advice' was to use twice weekly an oestrogen pessary as well as the oestrogen cream, and every night for one month a low-dose cortisone cream. Messy? Inconvenient? Maybe. But the results have been spectacular. My husband and I are back on track – enjoying regular, pain-free (or very minimal pain), lube-free, enjoyable sex. **– ANNE**

Regardless of how long you have been in your relationship, Dr Elias says we need to be more honest about ... everything. 'Talk about what's worrying you about sex or your relationship, or other stresses you have in your life ... because you're not going to be able to enjoy sex and be turned on if you're stressed and tense. You need to be relaxed enough to get turned on.'

Sometimes you might not be in the mood – but it can also be that you're not into the person you're with.

Sarah* talked to us about the painful sex she endured with her now ex-husband. Their relationship wasn't great and neither was the sex. 'I remember we were having sex and he said to me, "You're grimacing! You could *look* like you're enjoying it."

'It was often painful. I wouldn't initiate sex because I had all these negative emotions around it. Every time we'd sort of enter into sex I would be really nervous that something was gonna go wrong that he wouldn't be happy with ... and it would sometimes go for 45 minutes. I would want it to finish, especially when it was painful! ... Again I got in trouble – like, "Oh, you're looking at the clock! Come on, you should be enjoying it!"

'I wasn't attracted to him at that time, even though we were married. It was a lubrication issue as well. Not being attracted. Not being relaxed and not being happy. So it was just so painful.'

Sarah got out of that marriage and discovered that she could get wet – easily! – when her heart, head and body were in it. When she could do it with the right guy, who showed the right consideration, care and general sexiness, she had a blast. In a heartwarming song of sisterhood solidarity, her friends literally SCREAMED DOWN THE PHONE IN DELIGHT when she told them about her hot post-divorce sex.

Sex educator Emily Nagoski wants to communicate one important message to as many people as possible: **it is possible for your body to have signs of physical arousal and for you not to be sexually aroused.**

In her 2018 Ted Talk 'The truth about unwanted arousal', Dr Nagoski explains that you can have increased blood flow to your genitals in response to any sex-related stimuli, even if it's something that you don't want or like. Even if the stimuli is an assault or rape. You can be wet and engorged AND have your brain telling you, 'I don't want this'. When this happens, listen to your brain.

If you find yourself in a situation where you are showing signs of physical sexual arousal but you don't want to keep going – STOP. Tell the person you are with to listen to your words.

And don't let anyone tell you that your body knows better than you do.

There are many health conditions that can lead to painful sex, Remember vaginismus and vulvodynia, mentioned earlier in the chapter?

Vaginismus happens when pelvic floor muscles tighten and cause the vagina (which typically relaxes with sexual stimulation) to spasm involuntarily. This can create a feeling of tightness in the vagina that can make sexual penetration, Pap smears and even inserting a tampon painful ... if not impossible. The main causes of vaginismus include:

* ★ trauma or injury from childbirth or surgery
* ★ past sexual abuse, rape or trauma
* ★ endometriosis
* ★ tight pelvic floor muscles
* ★ recurring urinary tract infections
* ★ undiagnosed thrush
* ★ fear (of sex, pregnancy, sexual abuse, rape or the vagina being too small for sex)

Vaginismus triggered by feelings of fear, anxiety or stress is sometimes described as 'a panic attack of the pelvic floor'. Stress and anxiety can cause muscle tension in the pelvic floor in the same way that it can happen in any other part of the body.

> I experienced painful sex for years and as a dating woman this really affected my ability to form relationships with men. I was told by my doctor when getting a Pap smear that 'it's normal and it's unlikely to change'. This was an older doctor who specialised in women's health!
>
> It wasn't until I became a physiotherapist and was having a conversation with a women's health physio colleague that I realised it was common! I reached out and had a few assessments and found out I had vaginismus. With her help and with dilator therapy, I now do not experience pain with sex! It took eight years of pain and my doctor giving me horrible advice before I stumbled across something that could help me! As a healthcare professional, I truly am so shocked at how poorly understood this area is and how many women suffer in silence! – **ANGIE**

Vulvodynia is chronic pain that affects the vulva. It may occur in just one spot, or different areas from one time to the next. It's not understood what causes it and there is no known cure.

But self-care combined with medical treatments can help bring relief – the problem is, it isn't always easy to access the medical care you need to get these treatments.

Frankie* has had vulvodynia since she first became sexually active about 20 years ago. She describes it as having a 'temperamental vagina' and believes it is far more prevalent than many realise. 'It's also a condition that people shouldn't feel ashamed or embarrassed to talk about,' she says.

'It causes pain in my vulva and my vagina, particularly in relation to sex, but also in relation to things as innocuous as trying to insert a tampon. Adding to the frustration is the fact that if I'm having a day where my vulva really hurts, it's not something I can turn to a colleague and say, "I'm sorry, I'm a bit impatient today because of my vulva."'

Frankie still doesn't know why she suffers from vulvodynia and sometimes feels as though her body has betrayed her. None of this has been helped by the terrible experiences she's had with medical professionals, who have been dismissive of her pain and don't appreciate the impact it has had on her life.

Over the years Frankie has been prescribed everything from lubricants to different condoms, pain medication, treatment for chronic thrush, dilators, vibrators and sexual counselling. She describes it as an exhausting experience.

'It was actually the physiotherapy that proved most beneficial for me because that was the one that provided me with a better sense of how my body was working, and what was actually going on with my vulva and my vagina,' she says.

As is so often the case with women's health issues, getting a diagnosis if you have vaginismus or vulvodynia can be a difficult process.

Dr Elias says some doctors still aren't even aware of what vaginismus and vulvodynia actually *are*.

'Even some gynaecologists, I dread to say. So if someone thinks they might have this problem and they go to their doctor and the doctor says, "Oh, no, there's nothing wrong with you," then I'd like your readers to say to the doctor, "Are you familiar with vaginismus? Are you familiar with vulvodynia? And if not, please refer me to someone who is."'

When it comes to vaginismus, a good GP will try to treat physical symptoms of a dry vagina first to potentially reduce pain, which may decrease any fear. But if not, this is where a pelvic floor physio can help, and in some cases you might even require the support of a sex therapist.

Pelvic floor physio Angela James describes the vagina as being like a sock that sits flat until there is a foot inside it. 'It should be able to open when something goes inside, like a speculum, tampon or penis. But if that muscle is too tight, it loses its ability to expand, and it will often create pain, or the inability to even tolerate any penetration.'

Sometimes the muscle can be so spasmed, and has been for so long, that it has actually lost its ability to expand at all. When this happens, James can't do a vaginal assessment on a woman's first visit.

'The women are often very distressed, so they can present with years of not being able to tolerate a tampon, a finger, a penis, and no way a Pap smear. They've developed a trauma response so that their body's conditioned to expect pain, their muscles are so vigilant, and they're so protective.

'That's a really sad place for a woman to be because it stops her moving forward into things like relationships, or entertaining the thought of having a family. It really affects women at the heart of who they are.'

But here's the great thing. James says she can often help these women achieve their goal of being able to tolerate sexual intercourse, toys or a cervical screening test (which have replaced Pap smears). 'We address it like any other muscle, but we need to address it in a more sensitive nature because it's internal. We do a lot of education so that the problem makes sense. Once the problem makes sense, the fear dissipates. That's the first thing. Then we meet the woman with where she's at. How much can she tolerate? We just gradually push that further and further until she achieves her goal.'

Tanya is a gay woman in her early 30s with vaginismus and vulvodynia. She has found ways to enjoy sex. 'When two women have sex, there's more dialogue. You talk about what you want. If it's a casual encounter, I'm not necessarily going to say, "I have vaginismus," and go through my entire medical history, I might just say, "I'm not into penetration," and the sexual encounter can go on.

'Sometimes it's such a big turn-off that the encounter ends there. It's too uncomfortable and I'm no longer turned on and I don't want to keep having sex. I might say something like, "Can we stop?" ... Other times it's just about stopping and repositioning, or stopping and talking, asking to do something else in bed ... Rethinking the encounter.

'The person I am with and I – we both know that sex shouldn't be painful unless you want it to be. Having come out as gay and having to experiment and come up with a new script, gay women challenge this narrative that sex is meant to be painful. Women that I'm seeing, women in their 30s, aren't buying into this idea that sex is painful for women "naturally" or inherently.'

There are other health conditions that can lead to painful sex.

Michelle describes the pain she experiences during sex as being like 'someone stabbing a knife up my bowel'. Michelle isn't just experiencing pain during sex – she has endometriosis and lives with pelvic pain every day. But penetrative sex is definitely one of the most painful things she does.

'Sometimes I have panic attacks at the thought of having penetrative sex or sex in general because my mind knows it's going to lead to penetration.'

For a long time, Michelle thought her pain was just part of being a woman. When she finally talked to GPs about her symptoms, her experience wasn't validated. 'A lot of them said it was in my head or that they didn't really understand pain because it can be quite a complex topic.'

If painful sex is becoming a regular thing, please go see a GP (see the end of the chapter for how to get the most from that conversation). And remember that you are the expert when it comes to your own body!

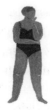

OTHER HEALTH CONDITIONS KNOWN TO CAUSE PAINFUL SEX

Beyond vaginismus and vulvodynia, there are a range of conditions that can contribute to painful sex. These are broadly broken down into two categories: those that cause entry pain at the vagina, and those causing pain deep in the pelvis.

Some illnesses or conditions of the pelvis that can cause pain deep inside the vagina during intercourse include:

- ★ endometriosis
- ★ cystitis
- ★ irritable bowel syndrome
- ★ pelvic inflammatory disease
- ★ ovarian cysts
- ★ adenomyosis
- ★ uterine prolapse and fibroids

Certain sexually transmitted infections (STIs) can lead to painful sex.

- ★ chlamydia
- ★ gonorrhoea
- ★ genital warts
- ★ herpes sores

The skin of your vulva is very delicate and extremely sensitive. When the skin on your vulva is **irritated, inflamed or infected**, it can cause painful intercourse. Certain conditions affecting the vulva, or part of it, can cause swelling, burning, itching, cracking, splitting, whitening, redness or discharge.

★ psoriasis
★ eczema
★ thrush
★ contact dermatitis
★ lichen sclerosus
★ lichen planus

Some medical treatments or surgery can also make sex painful.

★ hysterectomies
★ vaginal repairs for prolapse
★ episiotomies (the cut between the vaginal open and anus women sometimes get when they are giving birth)
★ chemotherapy
★ radiation therapy

Certain common medications can cause vaginal dryness in some women, which, without the right amount of lube and foreplay, can cause painful sex. You should always make sure you keep the consumer medicine information leaflet when you take medication, as it will highlight any side effects.

★ common cold and flu medication
★ anti-anxiety meds
★ some types of contraception

I just wanted to say thank you for the latest ep about painful sex. I have lichen sclerosus, a skin condition that causes tears in my vagina, which obviously makes sex very painful. I've also developed vaginismus as a result. I learnt some things from the episode but it mainly just helped me feel not so alone! – **ELLEN**

There is something we need to ask ourselves: why do we proceed with penetration and participate in sexual activities in spite of the pain?

'There's actually a lot of pride in a woman's ability to "take it" – whether it's in childbirth and not using drugs or whatever,' says Lili Loofbourow. 'Even our language about sex is, you know, "pounding", "slamming" or "banging" – and these terms lay the groundwork for sex to be uncomfortable or painful for women, and that that's just how it is,' says Loofbourow.

She reckons most men are fairly oblivious to the compromises that women make for the male orgasm. 'I don't think most men are monsters who want to be hurting the women they're having sex with. But the fact is, I think that's happening more than we realise.'

Dr Elias says she is seeing more women for painful sex than she used to, and her sense is that young women especially are under pressure to have types of intercourse they're not into.

'If they think that to get a partner, or keep a partner, you've got to have sex, and also have sex in ways that they may not particularly like, then naturally you're not going to get turned on.

'There's more of a demand for anal sex from their partners. But not only that, even with vaginal sex there's more aggressive or rough sex that's going on, because that's also seen in porn.'

Again, ladies, we need to talk about porn and its influence on our sex lives, sexuality, pleasure and wellbeing.

If you read erotic fiction written BY WOMEN, you'll notice there's as much focus on women's pussies being wet as there is on blokes having big hard dicks. This is not what you see in mainstream porn, where, to be blunt, the pussies we've seen look ... quite *dry*. And unaroused. Problem is, this is the same porn that teenagers watch – and it's often where they learn about sex. It's conditioning women and their partners to want sex that may not turn them on or may cause them pain.

Loofbourow sees it this way: 'For a lot of women, there are other pay-offs to sex like feeling close or intimate with your partner, or making someone else feel good. A lot of women are socialised to locate their pleasure in someone else's.

'The way that women are encouraged to self-present in order to be sexually attractive actually involves a fair amount of suffering: high heels wrench the body, so do corsets, and so do bras. I mean, there's a lot of routine discomfort that women are encouraged to ignore as they pursue romantic lives.'

Painful sex fits this overall pattern that we're expected to endure a good deal of discomfort if we want to attract and secure a male partner. 'It's hard to figure out where to draw that line when you're trained your whole life to please other people and to take pleasure in the fact that they find you pretty or attractive,' says Loofbourow. 'I think that can leave some people without the resources to recognise that they are literally in pain.'

But guess what? YOU HAVE THE RIGHT TO CALL 'STOP'. Because sex should never be painful.

Once more for the people up the back?

Sex should NEVER be painful.

Here's some ideas on how to call 'stop' on painful sex:

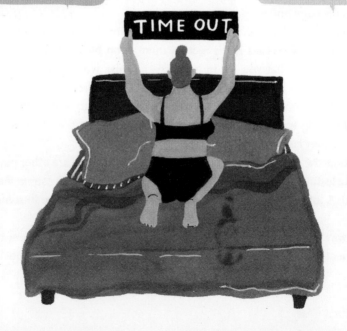

And some ideas on how to slow things down so that your body has time to get wet and warmed up:

I really want to take time on foreplay today! Let's go slow. It's my birthday.

I read this thing where a sex therapist suggested setting a timer so you don't rush straight to penetration. You wanna try it? Fifteen minutes? No dick until the timer sounds, OK?

I need more time to feel it. Can you feel this? Yeah, nothing. Slow down!

Hang on, I'm not even wet yet. What's the rush?

I'm just enjoying this for now. Can we do it a bit longer?

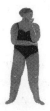

HOW TO TALK TO YOUR GP ABOUT PAINFUL SEX

OR ANY OTHER ISSUES YOU FEEL AWKWARD ABOUT

Give yourself a break. You're allowed to feel stressed or anxious about having this conversation. It's personal and it's real to you.

Call ahead. You can find out whether your doctor specialises in this field before stepping inside the clinic by calling reception and asking something like, 'I need to see a doctor about painful sex. Do you have someone there who knows about this?' Reception staff tend to be unflappable. Plus, it's over the phone so it's less confronting and it may save you an unnecessary visit to a doctor who is crap. (Reception staff LOVE to refer their best doctors.) If you already have a preferred doctor, you can ring or email ahead to give them a heads-up on the reason you'll be presenting at their clinic, and you can even warn them that you're feeling uncomfortable or nervous about what's coming.

Write notes. Have a list of everything you want to say so that if the words flee your head, you have a piece of paper to unfold, smooth on your lap and read from. (This can also be done on your smartphone.) Keep the list close by and add to it as specific things occur to you in the lead-up to your appointment. By the time you get there, you will feel prepared.

Know what you want to say and picture yourself saying it. Does this sound dorky? Great! It works, and used in conjunction with the last step, it will set you up to succeed.

Bring up the problem early in your appointment. Pretty much the moment you sit down, say something like, 'I wanted to see you because sex is getting painful for me.' Don't save it up. Allow the problem the time and attention it deserves.

It's OK to bring someone if you want. If your partner wants to come to the appointment and offer moral support, or even lead the conversation, that could be helpful. Or you could bring your partner or friend to wait in reception for you. It's completely OK to ask them to wait outside. And it's completely OK for you to say to your partner, 'Actually, I want to do this alone,' even halfway through the consultation.

It will get real. Be prepared to be asked personal questions and to be honest in your answers. There can be a bit of a 'visiting the school principal's office' vibe to seeing a doctor sometimes, but remember, you're not in trouble and there are no right or wrong answers.

Don't be put off. There are plenty of great GPs and women's health professionals out there, no doubt about it. But we have heard far too many stories of women not being listened to, which makes it hard for us to confidently say 'you should always listen to your GP'. So if you are not happy with how things are going with your GP – if they are dismissing you, telling you that your experience is all in your head, that it is just part of being a woman – go and find someone else. Get a second opinion. Or third.

You're the boss. In all matters to do with your body, you are the boss. Whether it's taking recommended medication, getting the doctor to believe you, leaving an uncomfortable situation, or choosing to stop sex that hurts, no-one can override your wishes. It's YOUR body, and you are the CEO, Boss, Prime Minister and Sovereign Leader of this body!

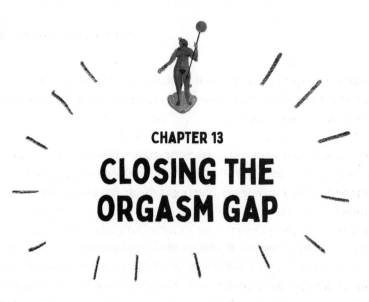

CHAPTER 13

CLOSING THE ORGASM GAP

Picture this: you and your partner have just had (hetero) sex. He came, and you didn't. He's finished. You're not. What's the best way to describe how you feel?

1. Totally fine – you came twice this morning when he went down on you before you got out of bed.
2. Relieved – he'd been pounding away for 20 minutes and you just wanted it to be over.
3. Silently furious – this happens all the time and you're sick of it.
4. Ready – as you hand him your vibrator.

We had never heard of the orgasm gap before the release of data from the Second Australian Study of Health and Relationships in 2014. But even though we may not have known the term, any heterosexual woman could have vouched for its existence.

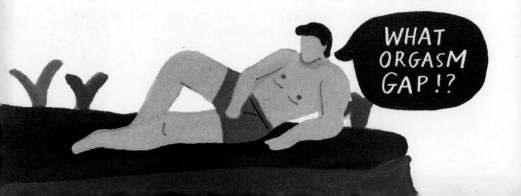

Between October 2012 and November 2013, researchers randomly called thousands of people between the ages of 16 and 69 and asked 20,094 of those who answered a suite of questions about their sex lives. This was a once-in-a-decade opportunity to take a good, hard look at what is going on in our sex lives. One of the many findings of Australia's most important study of sexual and reproductive health was that **92 per cent of men and 66 per cent of women had an orgasm during their most recent hetero sexual encounter**. That difference of 26 per cent? That's the orgasm gap. It's even bigger than the gender pay gap – and it's not closing any time soon.

Most of them wouldn't ask if I came. They would just be like, 'That was great,' give me a kiss goodnight and we were done. Or if they did ask, I would say something like, 'Oh, no I didn't, but that's OK,' and they would say, 'OK then,' and we were done. I suppose deep down I didn't want them to feel like they had to put in any extra effort for me, because it would take longer to get me off than them, which now in hindsight is so ridiculous. – **SOFIA**

So, what's the deal? Why do straight women strike out so drastically when it comes to orgasms?

Dr Melissa Kang says the findings of the Australian sexual health study are not unique. 'An even larger study in the US of over 50,000 people found a similar gap. In fact, it was bigger – about a 30 per cent difference.'

That US study posed a slightly different question and found that orgasms during sexual encounters were *usually* or *always* experienced by:

★ 95 per cent of heterosexual men
★ 89 per cent of gay men
★ 88 per cent of bisexual men
★ 86 per cent of lesbian women
★ 66 per cent of bisexual women
★ 65 per cent of heterosexual women.

To translate? Heterosexual women are the demographic having the fewest orgasms during sex.

Ladies, we need to talk about the ORGASM GAP.

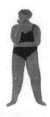

WHAT HAPPENED IN YOUR MOST RECENT SEXUAL ENCOUNTER?

There were lots of other amazing bits of data that came out of this particular question in the Second Australian Study of Health and Relationships, including some interesting differences in what men and women reported. Here's what researchers were told when they asked hetero men and women about their most recent sexual encounters:

- ★ 75 per cent had sex with a live-in partner, 17 per cent with a regular partner they did not live with, and 6.5 per cent with a casual or occasional partner.
- ★ 92.4 per cent of people had vaginal intercourse.
- ★ 82 per cent of men and 73 per cent of women reported manual stimulation of the woman by the man.
- ★ 71 per cent of men and 70 per cent of women reported manual stimulation of the man by the woman.
- ★ 31 per cent of men and 23 per cent of women reported cunnilingus (man's mouth on woman).
- ★ 27 per cent of men and 24 per cent of women reported fellatio (woman's mouth on man).
- ★ 1.2 per cent of men and 0.4 per cent of women reported anal intercourse.
- ★ 92 per cent of men had an orgasm and 66 per cent of women had an orgasm. (We know we've told you this before, but it's worth repeating.)

Are you seeing the pattern we're seeing here? There also seems to be a PERCEPTION GAP between what men and women are reporting.

The benefits of sharing orgasms with your partner are huge. If a woman orgasms, she experiences increased commitment, bonding and tolerance of imperfections in the relationship. Orgasms help us to care more about the wellbeing of our partner. And best of all? A good orgasm will motivate us to want sex AGAIN.

Tanya Koens is a sexologist and fierce fighter for everyone's right to enjoy sex who believes we all deserve acceptance, reassurance and our fair share of the orgasm cake.

Koens says women's chances of orgasms with a partner tend to get better the longer they are together. At the other end of the relationship spectrum – casual sex and one-nighters – things are pretty grim. 'I've seen **studies about hook-up sex where 55 per cent of men say they've had an orgasm, but only a measly 4 per cent of women**, which I'm totally dismayed at.'

She's not the only who's dismayed about this. Isn't the point of hook-up sex to have fun and, at least some of the time, have great sex?

> I took him back to my place, we were pashing, the clothes came off, then he flipped me over and I thought, 'Yes, love a man who takes control', then he hooked his arms under my armpits and up over my shoulders, looked me in the eyes and said, 'Are you ready?' I thought, 'OMG! Great! What's about to happen! Woot woot!' Then he jackhammered me for 30 secs, and oooh, it was over. I had a wet patch on my thigh. Didn't even enter me. – **TAYLOR**

Before we go any further, there's another thing Koens was able to confirm. The idea that the female orgasm is elusive and difficult? It's complete BOLLOCKS. When left to our own devices (masturbation), it takes women the same amount of time to get off as men.

'I've seen statistics of global surveys and from insertion of penis into vagina, it's about five-and-a-half minutes for men to ejaculate. Women need about 17 minutes on average of stimulation during partnered sex. For the research on time to orgasm when masturbating? For men it's four minutes, for women it's four minutes.

'That made me upset. I was like, "Why is this happening?" And I think it's because women and men don't understand how women's bodies work and how they arouse and then women get blamed. We're not teaching people or learning what works for us.'

We'll get to this shortly, but while we're speaking of gaps, can we talk about the perception gap?

Imagine you're having one of those confidential chats with a good mate, knowing no one can overhear. Your friend is on the verge of tears telling you that she's started dreading sex with her fella. She made the mistake of faking it early on and now she doesn't know how to tell him she doesn't like the sex they have.

You listen patiently, topping up her tea and making her laugh with your own stories of unsatisfying sex. Maybe you snatch her phone and subscribe to this great podcast called *Ladies, We Need To Talk*?

A few days later, YOUR fella happens to run into the bloke in question. Being an ally, he susses out if this guy is interested in going to some kind of massage workshop as a sort of male bonding thing.

But the bloke can't help himself ... he boastfully tells your fella that he's been reading up on the G-spot and trying new positions that will help him and his partner get off at the *same time*. He knows EVERYTHING about sex. He's seen some cool stuff in porn he'll probably convince her to try. He's starting from a high base, though: he already knows that she comes every single time they have sex.

Koens has spoken to many men over the years who have had no idea that

1. most women won't orgasm during penis in vagina sex,
2. many women fake it,
3. and this could actually happen on their watch.

It's a common case of perception being so far from reality that they may well be speaking Japanese to a platypus. 'They're assuming that it's all about the P-in-V sex,' says Koens.

'I've seen research that about 30 per cent of men think that all women will orgasm from intercourse.'

It can come as a shock to learn that this is NOT the case. 'I have so many men saying, "All of my previous girlfriends came that way." And I have to say, "Well ... *some of them might have been acting.*"'

I had literally just broken up with my gorgeous BF and this guy talked a big game about knowing how to please a lady and prided himself on giving multi-orgasms ... But nope, not a clue what to do when he went down on me. I almost burst out laughing and almost cried at the same time! Then he climbed up, rolled over, I started giving him head ... and he almost exploded after five secs, then pulled me up onto him. I was starting to feel the build as I was grinding him hard, he starfished me, then he suddenly came and ... I think he thought I came too? He said, 'That was amazing.' I was IN SHOCK. — **SLOANE**

✳ ✳ ✳

OK, we're going to try and put something to bed (yes, intended), once and for all. It's something we touched on (yes, intended) when we were looking at the clitoris: the notion that the vaginal orgasm is SUPERIOR to the clitoral orgasm.

This, friends, is bullshit.

The sex we see, in porn or mainstream culture, shows women having wonderful performative orgasms while their partner pounds away at their vaginas, like a train entering and leaving a tunnel on a nightmarish loop. There's very little foreplay. Very little genital stimulation. Very little oral sex. And the clitoral touch, if any, is rough, wrong and way too quick.

This is not how pleasure goes for most women. Women's bodies are different to men's and what gets us off is different. As we discussed in chapter 2, for the vast majority of people with a clitoris, the place where we experience the most pleasure is ... the clitoris. And it's not 'cheating' to do what you need to do to stimulate your clitoris (using hands, sex toys, mouth).

The vagina is much less sensitive. Even the G-spot, the mythical area on the front wall of the vagina, is believed to be a source of pleasure because it is part of the clitoral network, known by researchers as the clitourethrovaginal (CUV) complex, which mostly sits inside your pelvis. So, if you or your partner want to do your bit to close the orgasm gap, start with the clitoris.

Still don't believe us? Then believe the 2017 US study from the *Journal of Sex & Marital Therapy* that found **only 18 per cent of women were able to orgasm through penetrative sex**.

Or Dr Kang, who also references the Second Australian Study of Health and Relationships: 'The number one most likely cause of an orgasm for a woman was if it didn't actually involve penetrative intercourse.'

What *were* the sexual activities that made women orgasm? At the top of the list were having someone touch their genitals with their hands, oral sex, or a combination of the two.

Here's the kicker though: some of us can be quite uncomfortable about having our partners go down on us.

Koens says it's because we get a lifetime of bad press about our genitals. 'A lot of women don't feel very comfortable having someone's head right there in their personal bits because all their life they've been told that they don't look good, smell good, taste good.

They feel like apologising. It's like, "Oh my god, I'm sorry I didn't shave", "I didn't wax", "I don't smell good", "Oh, you've been on there for ages, should I send you a snorkel?"'

Dr Kang saw this come up a lot with Dolly Doctor over the years with readers saying, 'Oh, I don't want him to go down there. I don't want him to see me, to smell me.'

So, how do we start changing this?

'It's so hard to advocate for yourself when you've grown up your whole life being told that your job is to give men pleasure,' says Dr Kang. 'We need to start taking responsibility and advocate for ourselves. However, there's a lot of forces working against us.'

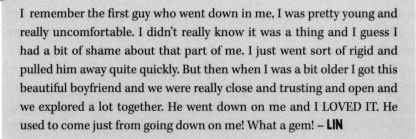

I remember the first guy who went down in me, I was pretty young and really uncomfortable. I didn't really know it was a thing and I guess I had a bit of shame about that part of me. I just went sort of rigid and pulled him away quite quickly. But then when I was a bit older I got this beautiful boyfriend and we were really close and trusting and open and we explored a lot together. He went down on me and I LOVED IT. He used to come just from going down on me! What a gem! – **LIN**

This book is just one small force pushing in the opposite direction. We thought a great way to convince women that their bodies and particular

THEIR VULVAS (yes, we're shouting) are NOT DISGUSTING and DON'T STINK was to hand the mic over to people who know.

'I used to be a stripper,' says Annie. 'I am 1000 per cent NOT advocating for becoming a stripper to get over your body issues, my god. But once you see how desperate and grateful they are to catch even a glimpse of a pussy, it really does sort of confirm that there can't be anything too repulsive about them!"

And you know who else knows about pussies? Lesbians.

'I think back on the vaginas I've growled out and I remember every vagina tasted amazing,' says Ali. 'Of course it's cerebral – if you want someone, you want them everywhere, especially in your mouth.'

All the lesbians we talked to around this were a little nonplussed by the question.

'As a gay woman, my thinking around pussy is just so unconscious,' said Ali. 'Sure, the first time you do it, you might be nervous (smells, tastes) and that's natural, but I have never been worried about my flaps or the "look" of my vagina. I just don't think it's an issue. In fact I've never even heard queers talk about it (shape, form) – ever! That must be significant.

'I mean it's such an intimate act – and it's glorious. There are a million uses for your tongue and you get to find out what works and there's nothing more thrilling than having a woman arch her back as you're going down on her.'

DJ Sveta found herself embraced by the queer/kink scene from an early age, and it was a place where openness and acceptance were super normal. 'In my many years on being alive as a woman (albeit with extremely limited experience with cis straight men), I have never come across a man who is grossed out by pussies, nor have I heard any instances like that from any of my female friends.

'My advice to straight women would be to work on their self-esteem, meet far more sex-positive people, dump any man who would actually ever allude to such a thing and question whether those men are actually straight.'

Candy wanted to send a message to anyone who might be grossed out by their own vulva. 'Perhaps try eating a mango slowly or squishing through mochi or devouring a fig … This disgust, this self-hatred is so learnt, so taught – unlearn it. Get some water-based lubricant and explore … Female orgasm is the hill I will die on and only you can bring yours to fruition!'

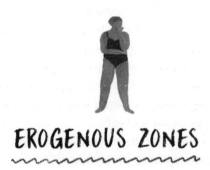

EROGENOUS ZONES

Your erogenous zones are parts of the body that are especially sensitive. When you touch or stimulate these tingly pleasure zones, you can feel relaxed, become aroused, experience pleasure, and sometimes orgasm.

Remember, what works for one person may not work for another. Those tiny little ear nibbles that seem to send electric signals to your clitoris can annoy the hell out of the next person. But here are some of the common erogenous zones known to get women going:

★ around the genital area, including the clitoris (inside and outside the pelvis), urethral opening, vaginal opening, perineum and anus
★ labia and inner thighs
★ breasts and areola

Then there are the completely non-sexual body parts that can be highly erotic for some people. We're talking about ears, back, neck, hands, thighs, back of the knees, wrist, mouth and scalp.

And let's not forget our brains. Even if your brain isn't technically an erogenous zone, it plays a vitally important role when it comes to getting ready for pleasure.

The best way to understand where your erogenous zones are is for you to explore. You can do it with your partner and that can be a lot of fun.

You will probably discover that intention can make a huge difference to the way touch is received. Take, for instance, your armpits. Being touched there by a friend can be extremely tickly, so much so that you're screaming and wriggling away. But a sports physio getting his fingers in there can be completely UNtickly – you receive the touch calmly and it's weirdly neutral. A parent or child caressing your neck will feel completely different to an intimate partner doing it, and your body will respond differently. Yes, mind and body are impossible to disentangle.

Self-touch can be delightfully pleasurable but also different to erotic touch from another. The advantage of exploring your erogenous zones by yourself is that the next time you connect with another person, you're going to be in the perfect position to let your partner know exactly what you like and how you'd like it. Your body, you get to decide.

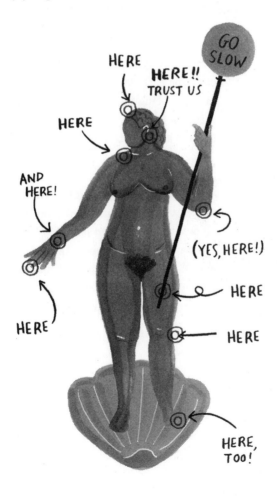

If you're perfectly happy with your sex life as it is and you're feeling in sync with your partner(s), that's AMAZING. Keep going. Have fun. Send us a postcard!

But one of the shortcomings of the sexual model we pick up over the course of our lives is that we are expected to flick a switch and be immediately turned on. Or we're meant to go through some fairly perfunctory foreplay – a quick pash, a tit squeeze, a rub on the thighs – and move quickly to penetration.

Koens says most of us need to walk down a long and sensual path before we get anywhere near P-in-V penetration. 'It's *all about* warming up. It's about experiences. It's about genital stimulation, it's about oral sex, it's about kissing. These things can get left out when people are in a hurry.

'When I speak to couples, quite often they're in a big hurry to get to P-in-V. I'm always like, "Why are you in a hurry to get to dessert? What about the entree? What about the main meal?"'

Listen to this wise woman. SLOW DOWN. Spend more time on foreplay. Don't rush. Foreplay, in case this isn't clear, doesn't even have to involve any touching. It's about connecting, being intimate and focusing on the person you are with. Koens likes to call foreplay 'outercourse', because that doesn't imply that something is coming afterwards. It is an activity in and of itself.

My top foreplay move would be sitting on your bed with your vibrator, having the time of your life. With your partner over the other side of the room, not allowed to touch, not allowed to play, just having to watch. Keep going as long as you want, teasing them. And then let them join you when you feel like it. It just drives them crazy, because they want what they can't have. They enjoy seeing you get off and they're just thinking about what they're gonna have soon. I am the object of desire.
– GEORGIA

We're going to come back to something that we've spoken about often in this book: knowing your body. And in this case, this means knowing *what turns you on* and *what types of touch you enjoy.*

For a lot of us, it takes until middle age to feel comfortable experimenting on our own or with partners. Same-sex couples are much better at figuring this out earlier than their hetero pals and a lot of the research points to this being because their sexual model isn't so prescribed. Pop culture and porn haven't laid down such immovable expectations, so they have to make their own way. Straight people could learn a lot from that.

Depending on the girl, or the mood, it can be quite a sexy and sensual thing. Soft, slow kisses, fingertips up the stomach to the breasts and tickles on the inner thigh, behind the knee, or massages to the calves and feet. Or it can be like a savage attack like you haven't eaten in days and you're just going at it.

A lot of people kind of focus on what they're doing with their mouth and are so focused on the clitoris, hitting that spot. They forget that there's a whole other body. Hitting all those other zones, the stomach, the nipples, the inner arms, the inner thighs, the feet. You have your hands free to explore a whole body.

I remember a time when I was receiving some really good head. The girl just had her hands all over my body. She was listening to my sound. She was feeling my movements. She was touching me in all the right places. – **JESSIE**

It doesn't have to go: kissing, touching, undressing, penis in vagina, thrust-thrust-thrust, finish. Whether or not orgasms are a priority, you can do things YOUR OWN WAY.

And much as we are loath to cloud your imagination with our suggestions, it *could* go something like: kissing, touching, undressing, kissing, licking, massage, neck kissing, licking, nibbling, fingering, licking and fingering, orgasm, kissing, go back for seconds, massage, head rubs, licking, P-in-V, sucking, OMG, orgasm, nigh nigh, zzzzzz …

In the last chapter we looked at physical arousal: increased heart rate, nipples hardening, vulva and vagina becoming engorged and wet. This is important for you to have physically enjoyable sex, the kind that doesn't hurt and the kind that can lead to orgasm (if you want).

But even more important is being turned on mentally, where you know you want sex. You're thinking about it. You're titillated, hot for it, warming up.

Once I had this thing with a guy. We got in this weird messaging each other thing ... It started kind of fun and innocent, playful flirting, and then got pretty fkn hot. It went on for MONTHS. I was a walking erection. I actually had to google if you could give yourself a yeast infection from being wet all the time (it's cool, you can't). I'll also add this though: our texts were sexy and sexually explicit, but I also felt seen by him, he thought I was funny, and he was interested in me and thought about me, you know, and it was horny as hell. – **SASS**

You should be BOTH mentally and physically aroused to be ready for sex. If you're not mentally ready, then it shouldn't happen. If you're not physically ready, then you shouldn't do it because you'll be signing up for sex that is unsatisfying or painful or both.

This brings us to DESIRE.

For a long time we have had this Hollywood idea of what horniness looks like – it's the *spontaneous desire* that comes over you when you see someone hot, you feel turned on and your body makes it pretty clear that you're horny.

Anyone can experience spontaneous desire, but the reality check is it does tend to be more common in men and much less so for women in longer-term relationships. You might experience it when you've been away from your partner for a couple of weeks and you reunite with some spontaneous hot sex.

Responsive desire, which tends to be the common experience for women in long-term relationships, is a term you may be less familiar with.

In the early 2000s, Canadian sex therapist Rosemary Basson published a paper called 'Rethinking Low Sexual Desire in Women', in which she argued that sexual desire isn't just about getting horny because your plumber made eye contact while jamming his thumb into a 15-millimetre copper pipe. It's a combination of factors that start with feeling safe and open to stimulation. What follows then are major components of women's sexual satisfaction: trust, intimacy, the ability to be vulnerable, respect, communication, affection and pleasure from sensual touching.

This kind of desire, which tends to be more common for women, especially those in longer-term relationships, doesn't just 'happen'. Responsive desire occurs when you *create the right environment to become aroused*.

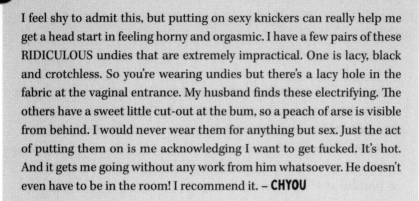

I feel shy to admit this, but putting on sexy knickers can really help me get a head start in feeling horny and orgasmic. I have a few pairs of these RIDICULOUS undies that are extremely impractical. One is lacy, black and crotchless. So you're wearing undies but there's a lacy hole in the fabric at the vaginal entrance. My husband finds these electrifying. The others have a sweet little cut-out at the bum, so a peach of arse is visible from behind. I would never wear them for anything but sex. Just the act of putting them on is me acknowledging I want to get fucked. It's hot. And it gets me going without any work from him whatsoever. He doesn't even have to be in the room! I recommend it. – **CHYOU**

Call it what you will – desire, libido, sex drive, horniness, eroticism, lust, pleasure – it's something that you don't tend to think about, until it goes away. And this is something that happens all too often for women over 40, according to Australian research published in 2017. Researchers from Monash University (including Dr Rosie Worsley from the hormones chapter) found that **70 per cent of women over 40 said that they lack sexual desire**.

The figure was so much higher than the researchers expected that they recommended GPs start routinely asking women about their libido.

Let's be clear, there is no 'right level' of desire, but when it's not matched to your partner's it can put a lot of pressure on your relationship. Not to mention the fact that good sex is AMAZING.

Once again our understanding of an issue has been centred around the male experience. So it's been assumed that the male libido is the norm, and anything that deviates from that experience is somehow defective. If a woman is not spontaneously aroused, then the perception has been that there must be a problem with *her* sex drive.

The truth is, women are more likely to experience spontaneous desire with a new partner or novel situation. Dr Basson's research into desire not only helped normalise the experience of many women who previously felt like there was something wrong with them, it also created an opportunity for those of us with a lower libido to think differently about desire and put us back in the driver's seat.

But it's not just about boredom and our need for novelty and adventure. There are a bunch of things that can affect your libido, and rarely is there a single cause.

Here are some that often come up:

* **hormonal variations:** different times in your cycle, pregnancy, breastfeeding, perimenopause or postmenopause
* **medication:** certain antidepressants and contraceptive pills
* **mental health:** depression, anxiety and other mental illnesses; trauma, stress and body dissatisfaction
* **painful sex:** dyspareunia, vaginismus or vulvodynia (as discussed in the previous chapter)
* **medical conditions:** feeling unwell; conditions such as endometriosis, prolapse, thrush, UTIs and pelvic diseases
* **life stuff:** being too busy, too tired or too overcommitted
* **relationship:** feeling pressured to have sex when you don't want to, being unhappy in your relationship, not being compatible, not having good communication and not feeling connected to your partner

Christina Spaccavento is a sex therapist and relationship counsellor, and in her clinical work she's found that women need more time to physically and emotionally connect with their partner to get ready for any kind of sexual interaction.

'I often say to my clients that it's OK, no-one has to push through – what we have to do is work around it. You can start from a place of feeling neutral. You can start from a place of willingness. "I don't feel turned on, I don't feel turned off."'

She encourages couples to create a space where they can connect. It's about taking the pressure off the less aroused partner, which also means being open to the fact that interactions might not end in penetrative sex or even any kind of sexual touching.

It can be really hard to talk to your partner about your needs for intimacy and to get away from the idea that foreplay needs to lead somewhere, that it needs to take you from A to B. Explaining this can be difficult.

Spaccavento says that one key to getting these conversations right is to talk outside of the heat of the bedroom. She's a big fan of 'couple chats', which require finding a time and place where you are going to have privacy and a few hours to talk – not a quick chat in the kitchen before you go to work.

'Bring your notebooks, sit down, and start to talk about what it is you like, what it is that you'd like to explore. This is the space where, if we're talking about the woman, she can say, "I need more time to connect with you," "I need to feel emotionally closer," "I'm not ready when you're ready," or "I need more touch in those areas of my body where I feel really good."

'It gives the partner the opportunity to listen first of all, to take on that advice. And then to try it out. It's actually at the deepest layer of intimacy. And what is another word for intimacy? Closeness ... What's another word? Connection ... What's another word? Vulnerability.

'We go to the most vulnerable places when we start to talk about the things that are most intimate to us. And that is often our sex life.'

Dr Anne-Frances Watson is a researcher who's studied sex education and how it affects young people and their sexuality.

Unsurprisingly, she found that our school sex ed is not great: young people are taught nothing about pleasure, nothing about female arousal and nothing about communication – the most essential things we need if we want to have partnered fun.

As a society we're not equipping youngsters with the information and tools they need to be able to navigate their sex lives in an informed, safe and empowered way. Basically, we're *not* setting people up for great sex.

'When you're starting out like that, then how are you going to get to a point where you're in bed, and you're like, "Oh, no, that's not doing it for me. Just move your hand down a little bit"?' asks Dr Watson.

'The only bit of advice young people seem to get about sex and communication is "you can say no". They're not told how to say yes. They're not told how to negotiate doing what they want to do.'

Dr Watson suggests we could learn something from some of the friendly fetishists in the kink community. 'The kink community is way ahead of the rest of us … Consent, boundaries, all of that kind of stuff, is discussed before you engage in sexual activity.

'I think young people really should be taught to *discuss* things before they *do* things. That is how you get pleasure. It's being able to say to somebody, "You know what? When you touch me here and you press down on that, that really does it for me."'

Remember Sofia from the start of the chapter? Well, she has successfully managed to close the orgasm gap.

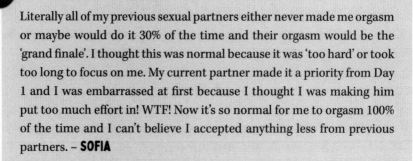

Literally all of my previous sexual partners either never made me orgasm or maybe would do it 30% of the time and their orgasm would be the 'grand finale'. I thought this was normal because it was 'too hard' or took too long to focus on me. My current partner made it a priority from Day 1 and I was embarrassed at first because I thought I was making him put too much effort in! WTF! Now it's so normal for me to orgasm 100% of the time and I can't believe I accepted anything less from previous partners. – **SOFIA**

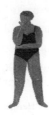

TOP 10 FOREPLAY TIPS FOR OUR PARTNER

When we asked the *Ladies, We Need To Talk* community to send us their top foreplay tips for partners, we were inundated with advice. We're sharing some of the popular tips with you here.

1. **Slow down.** Yep, we've already said it, and we'll say it again. The number one most popular foreplay tip from the podcast audience was to go slow.

2. **Forget everything you ever saw in porn.** It's safe to assume that pornography is a clear guide on how NOT to do it.

3. **Touch everywhere but the vulva.** Like the lag between ordering a pizza and the pizza arriving makes you absolutely GAG for that cheesy thin slice when it finally gets through your door – make her WANT it, but don't deliver too soon! It's often better to *delay* touching or giving any attention to the clitoris until after you've awakened other erogenous zones, so learn her erogenous zones. (Hot tip: they're not all 'rude' bits.)

4. **Tell your partner what you like about her.** Words can be extremely sexy. Use words to appreciate her, make her feel safe, make her feel wanted. This can start with text messaging before you even get in the same place. A plan of all the yummy things you hope to do together? These kinds of communications are often unspoken and so can be outrageously hot when said aloud.

5. **Don't be afraid to receive pleasure.** It's a form of surrender. And it's good.

6. **Oral is awesome.** Get it on a T-shirt. Oral is an art form and the best artists keep learning and practising their craft well into old age. If a woman feels apologetic or ashamed of her body, and the thought of you having your face down there makes her uneasy, it's brilliant if you can communicate how much you like it and want to be there. If being ears-deep in pussy is your happy place, tell her!

7. **Don't be afraid to show off.** Be silly. Be a food. Sex toys optional. Laughter essential.

8. **Take the pressure off yourself.** Don't be goal-oriented all the time. Yeah, this chapter is about orgasm, but not all touch has to lead to sex and not all sex has to lead to orgasm.

9. **Be vulnerable.** And if you're not sure what that means? It's basically the opposite of playing it cool. Be real. Expose your heart. *That's* living on the edge. And it can be super sexy.

10. **Show consideration to your partner.** When we asked for the favourite foreplay move your partner can do for you, this was high on the list. Be attentive, do the dishes, cuddle, touch and care. Put the kids to bed. Tidy up. Doing the chores that are usually her problem is MASSIVELY hot. And the experts we spoke to agree: foreplay begins the minute that sex ends.

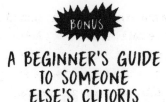

A BEGINNER'S GUIDE TO SOMEONE ELSE'S CLITORIS

1. **Relax and take your time.** This is not a race and it can distract her if she senses any impatience. Pleasuring someone's clitoris requires touch that is consistent, repetitive and ongoing, and it will need to go on for some time, so arrange yourself in a position that is comfortable for you.

2. **Gentle side-to-side touch is preferred.** Not scraping, but soft rubbing. If your partner wants more, they will probably tell you or indicate this nonverbally – but you're better off starting very gently. Our advice? If what you usually do is a 10? Try applying a 1 or a 2. Side-to-side stroking of the clitoris is usually preferred. Top-to-bottom stroking is also good, as is circular stroking, but bottom-to-top touch rarely feels good. It tends to hurt as it attacks the urethra (pee hole).

3. **Switch on your antenna to what your partner's body is trying to tell you**, especially if you feel unsure, inexperienced or unschooled. A lot of people involuntarily communicate their likes and dislikes. For example, if her thighs clamp together, whatever you're doing between her legs is too much, too forceful or unwelcome. If her legs open wider and she is thrusting towards you, she is liking what you're doing and you could probably stand to apply a little more pressure.

4. **If she is nearing orgasm, continue doing what you're doing**. Don't speed up or apply more pressure. Just hold firm, you're doing great.

5. **Immediately after orgasm the clitoris can feel terribly sensitive and you want to avoid touching it**, except very, very gently. But seriously? Maybe not at all.

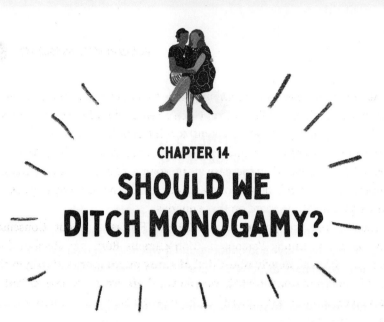

CHAPTER 14

SHOULD WE DITCH MONOGAMY?

We all know how it goes. Girl meets boy. They like each other enough to want to growl on each other's naughty bits. Something gets in the way, which leads to high drama. But they overcome the obstacles, fall in love again and spend the rest of eternity making out under flattering lighting and looking 25.

This story is *everywhere* in most cultures. So you can bet your nanna's false teeth it's had an influence on your romantic life. The message is pretty clear: one partner, one bed, one life. Same face every morning.

The only alternatives to this monogamy path are the sad and lonely path, which tends to involve cats, ice cream and misery, or the cheating path, where someone decides to bonk a person who is not their partner. That second option usually ends in tears – and the sad and lonely path.

But what if there are OTHER paths that we're missing here?

Sex therapist and relationships counsellor Desiree Spierings has had a lot more people coming to see her to discuss open relationships in recent years. She's not sure if it's because more people are exploring alternatives to monogamy or if they are just more willing to talk about it.

'There's more knowledge around it. I definitely feel we're more aware of the fact that relationships can look very different nowadays than what we used to think or were OK with.'

At the very least, we seem to want to know more about different relationship options. A US study of Google search data found an increasing number of people actively looking for information on alternatives to monogamy. Researchers examined Google Trends data for the period from 2006 to 2015 and found an increase in the volume of searches for terms such as 'open relationships', 'polyamory' and 'consensual non-monogamy', as well as the amount of time spent on these queries.

Then there's the paper from 2020 on 'Fantasies About Consensual Nonmonogamy Among Persons in Monogamous Romantic Relationships'. The research found **nearly one-third of study participants divulged that being in an open relationship was part of their favourite sexual fantasy of all time**, and the vast majority of these people said they wanted to act on this fantasy in the future.

Maybe ....we're not as committed as we thought we were?

Ladies, we need to talk about DITCHING MONOGAMY.

We are perfect for each other in literally every other aspect of our lives and bring out the best in each other. We are the ultimate BFFs. But the sex life just isn't fulfilling. My husband just doesn't dig sex that much, never has (apart from the honeymoon period where we were shagging ALL the time). I'm the opposite. I am really passionate about sexuality and pleasure.

My nan and pop were swingers for most of their married life. Maybe that's where my influence came from – my nan has always been very open about her sexual experiences and desires. She's still very much alive and dirty as ever.

The lack of sex for my husband and I has never been a huge issue in our relationship but the longer we are together, the less sex we have. We have discussed the topic (minimally) of opening our relationship in the hopes that it will bring back the spark in our sex life for both of us. Not seeking emotional connection, purely sexual.

I think our partnership is definitely strong enough but I just don't think we are quite there yet, and are too scared of the damage it could do to our otherwise perfect relationship and all the judgement we might receive. **–LASH**

For some women, the idea of wanting to cram MORE into our schedules is baffling. Even if that MORE is more sex, more love, or more pleasure – we're freaking busy! So why would we do it?

There's a lot of reasons why rejecting monogamy seems to be a growing trend. People in polyamorous and open relationships tend to report the lowest levels of jealousy, relatively high levels of relationship satisfaction and pretty much off-the-chart levels of sexual satisfaction.

As we know from the last chapter, female desire is complicated, and can become more so in a long-term monogamous relationship – 'not because women don't like sex, but because it's harder for them to be interested in sex with the same person over and over and over,' says Dr Wednesday Martin.

Dr Martin is an author, researcher and cultural critic with a background in anthropology. Her book *Untrue* collated international research and led her to challenge the idea that women are less horny than men.

'A sex researcher named Marta Meana interviewed women who reported low desire in their long-term relationships, and were distressed by it. They said, "I want to *want* my husband again!" And Meana said to them, "What would happen if you could have sex with a handsome and attractive stranger?" Women said, "Oh, are you kidding? My sexual desire would be back very quickly!" Women, at least as much as men, need variety and novelty and adventure.'

Based on what she has learnt in her research and with her clients, Meana argues that something about the roles women take on in relationships and their familiarity with their partners tends to stifle female desire.

Could it be that the cosy intimacy and safety of a long-term relationship isn't creating a space for women to feel safe and sexy, but rather the perfect environment for tedium and indifference? Dr Martin says she spoke to plenty of experts who told her that while hetero men in long-term relationships report being sexually satisfied, for women it is a very different story.

She found that in committed, long-term relationships, many women find their desire for their partners drops off dramatically between one and four years in. As for men? 'They are pretty happy having sex with their long-term partners for 9 to 12 years without courting boredom.'

That doesn't mean we're not having any sex at all with our partners. Even when we have no desire, we often decide to do it anyway. 'So you say, "I'm going to have sex for the team, for the good of the marriage, to placate my male or female partner." So then you start to have what we call "service sex",' says Dr Martin.

'There's nothing wrong with a maintenance shag once in a while – husbands do it for their wives sometimes. But service sex is something different. It's when it becomes a deeply ingrained habit and you lose sight of your entitlement to sexual pleasure of your own.

'I believe there is an epidemic of service sex - of women providing sex to their long-term male partners, without joy and without pleasure, and we absolutely have to stop it.'

Before she started writing her book, Dr Martin thought that it was men asking for polyamorous and open relationships so they could have more sex. But looking at the history of polyamory in the United States and worldwide, she quickly realised that her assumption, while common, was all wrong.

'It's women, by and large, who are the relationship revolutionaries coming in to therapists with their husbands or male partners and saying, "I want us to introduce a third into our relationship."'

And even when men introduce and encourage their female partners to engage in consensual non-monogamy, Dr Martin says it's often the female partner who wants to keep going.

'The expression is, once the genie is out of the bottle, she's not going back. Once women have the variety and novelty and adventure ... it is hard to give it up.'

Madeleine is 42 and met her partner when she was 18. 'I embarked on my career and was very taken up by that for about a decade, then children and was taken up by that for about five years. He knew that I was bisexual but it wasn't very pressing.'

Five years ago she decided that she wanted to be able to explore her queer identity. 'I sort of realised that I wasn't done. The queer part of myself needed some sort of expression or I was going continue to be miserable.'

Madeleine and her partner had a few years of talk before she decided that, yes, she wanted to be non-monogamous.

'The first time I had sex with a woman after all this time ... I felt really free, and it's corny to say, but I felt like I was coming into my power. It was a very exhilarating moment, quite scary too, because it's a gamble and a risk. You're kind of inhabiting this liminal space between institutions and society. You can feel divided. It's quite stressful. You're trying to get everything to work and keep all the balls in the air. But I can't go back to how it was.'

Madeleine is now seeing three women. 'We're all really honest about where we're at.'

'My partner and I don't have sex much, but we're warm with each other. We back each other. We hold hands when we're watching telly. We parent our kids together. It's almost like he's seen, "Madeleine needs to do this thing now, and I'm just going to wait and see what happens."

'ALL of my female friends are going through a questioning process. Their children are old enough that they have a bit more agency and they can put their heads up and go, "What do I want? How do I forge something that's better for me?"'

Desiree Spierings says people she sees who are considering open relationships are seeking intimacy and a deeper connection. They just want it with MORE THAN ONE PERSON. 'There is this misconception that it's kind of raunchy or very sexual. That is not the case. It's just like people who are in monogamous relationships, but with a few more people.'

Wendee, 50, is a swinger in a polyamorous relationship with two men.

'Ironically, I have less sex now than I did when I had only one partner! However, I have a much more fulfilling sex life now. I have a LOT more of the sex that I want to have than when I was in a monogamous relationship.

'In monogamy, you make a commitment to each other to not have sex with anyone else. So sometimes I consented to sex even if I wasn't really in the mood – even though I would often get into it eventually. In my current poly relationship, I don't feel the obligation to do that. I don't have sex for any other reason than because I want to and I feel like it.'

Stephanie is a 32-year-old trans woman who lives with what she calls her 'nesting partner'. She has two other longer-term partners.

'Honestly, the best part for me is having multiple partners with varying interests. Each of my partners is like an amazing friend that I have different things in common with, and each relationship fills a different need in my soul.

'My nesting partner is just the most caring, loyal person that I know, and I know she's got my back no matter what. Partner two is an amazing human who teaches me all of the things I missed out on because I never had a "female childhood". She finds joy in helping me with make-up and having sleepovers and she loves documenting the changes that oestrogen has made to my body. Partner three is my video game buddy who gives me part of the "typical female experience" that my other two partners can't (dating a man). He's really good at making me feel small and feminine and I need that sometimes.'

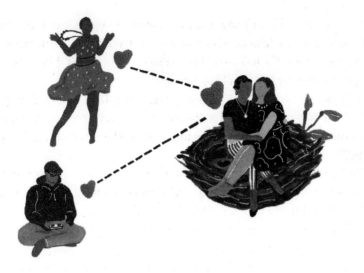

Stephanie adds, 'I think a lot of people assume that we're greedy. Which honestly is kind of true. I am poly because I'm greedy. I think there's multiple people out there that I'm capable of loving and I don't understand why I should limit that to one person.'

I am a healthy, fit, sexually active 60-year-old single woman (divorced after 31 years of marriage) now finding myself having sex with married men who are in open marriages, dating single men and being hit on by married men who aren't in open relationships (which I won't associate with). I have a more than platonic, sexual relationship with one open-married man and have met his wife three times. We have a great time as friends (no three-ways). While we have no interest in being together, he makes me happier than any other man I've ever been with.

I know most people would not only frown on all of this but be shocked, judgemental and probably shun me as a friend and a person. Yet the whole situation is opening me up sexually and making me much less needy of a serious, monogamous relationship. In fact, I think if I met someone that wanted to be in a relationship with me, he would have to be open to an open, polyamorous relationship. Am I crazy to be doing this at my age? I'm sure if my kids knew they would freak out ... which is probably what worries me the most. – **JERI**

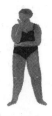

DIFFERENT TYPES
OF NON-MONOGAMY

Open relationship: A couple that is open to sexual experiences with people outside the relationship.

Consensual or 'ethical' non-monogamy: An arrangement where people explore love and sex with multiple people and everyone involved in the relationship(s) gives their consent.

Polyamory: Having more than one open romantic relationship at a time, where all parties give consent to there being more than one relationship.

Polygamy: This involves being married to more than one spouse at a time.

Swinging: Generally, casual sex without commitment.

Monogamish: 'A relationship that is mostly monogamous, but occasionally exceptions are made for sexual play,' according to the Urban Dictionary.

Don't ask, don't tell (DADT): A couple who agree to intimacy outside of the relationship, but don't share information about that intimacy with each other.

CONSENT is a concept that polyamorists frequently discuss.

'Sometimes there is this misconception about polyamory that, oh, it's just a leave pass to cheat, but it's really consented to,' says Spierings.

Stephanie agrees. 'I think a lot of people assume that we're more likely to cheat,' she says. 'My nesting partner and I communicate really well and I trust her absolutely, so I think she's actually less likely to cheat or leave than most people in a mono relationship.

'This is why the "ethical" part of ethical non-monogamy is really important to me. If you're totally open and communicate like adults then there's no reason for a poly relationship to have any less trust than a mono one.'

Imani* also puts open communication at the centre of her non-monogamous relationship. 'At first I thought I wanted "don't ask, don't tell", but there's a jealousy and anxiety in not knowing what's going on.

'Now we've landed at a place where we are not all up in each other's relationships, but we share what's happening, both practically and emotionally. We talk about our feelings really openly and frequently. We ask questions and reflect and answer honestly.

'I feel like many long-term relationships end because of situations precisely like what was brewing with us. There's dissatisfaction, then infidelity (we live in the world, there's always going to be sparks and connections with other people from time to time), then lies and hurt feelings. I feel so proud of us ... Feels like we beat the system.'

Rose* thought she was meeting a polyamorous Frenchman on a dating app. 'Poly' was clearly written on his profile. In real life he was handsome and the chemistry was genuinely wild. The romance that started off as a one-night stand ended up spanning three continents and more than three years.

But then Rose realised that the original premise under which they'd met ... was a lie.

'I was asking him questions about his life in Paris and about his family. And bit by bit, I suppose as he trusted me more and more, it became clear that he wasn't actually poly at all and that he and his partner were actually monogamous and he was cheating on her – which was quite a shock.

'Anyone can *say* they're polyamorous. And many people feel polyamorous and feel like, yes, I do fall in love with other people. And just because I love one person doesn't mean I love another any less. In the same way that you don't love one child less than their sibling or one friend less than another.

'The difference is there are many people out there practising polyamory and doing it honestly. So a huge aspect of it is honesty and consent. Consent is at the centre of the story.'

For a long time Shy followed the monogamy path: partner, two kids, big house. She described herself as the 'good girl that would cook up a storm and entertain and get the children to school and have her own businesses'.

But when her marriage broke down, she was drawn back to the kink scene she'd discovered in early adulthood and soon immersed herself in poly life.

'It definitely doesn't have to be sexual. What you find is that by connecting with different people, you're able to explore different parts of yourself. My partner isn't necessarily someone who I can get everything from. They can't be my everything. So then you realise you can make deeper connections. You can have sexual connections with other people and you can have all sorts of different connections with other people and start creating deeper, more intimate relationships.'

Not everyone will be into the kink play and interactions that Shy loves, but there's something appealing about the relationships she talks about where there is a focus on clear and respectful communication, and where consent reigns supreme and everyone's pleasure matters.

'I just had to go back to that place where I felt I could be myself. I felt so disconnected from everything and everyone. I just needed to go and find my people.'

Her people are those who let her be her AUTHENTIC self.

It's hard to have a non-monogamous lifestyle without a community that supports you. And experts are starting to realise that one very important factor in making polyamory work – or not – is culture and stigma.

Since breaking up with the Frenchman, Rose* has gone on to really embrace the poly community. She's done years of research into polyamory, read books and listened to podcasts. 'There's a really good support group. It's called Multiamory. It's a podcast and online forum as well.' She's also attended meetings with her current partner.

'To be honest, if I met someone who said they were part of the community but had demonstrated that they didn't care that much about consent or honesty or conversations or learning? I would doubt whether they were really polyamorous.'

Stephanie's mum struggled to come to terms with the way she lives.

'My mum has more issues with me being poly than she does with me being trans,' she says. 'She worries that my nesting partner will leave me or that I'm not the focus of their life. She just treats my nesting partner as though we're monogamous and goes quiet if I bring up anyone else. I'm not too fussed. I know my needs a lot better than she does. She has two failed marriages so I really don't understand why she feels that her values are the right ones. They've brought her a lot of unhappiness.'

Stephanie says it definitely helps to have friends who are part of the poly lifestyle.

'I don't really discuss any partner stuff at work. I worry about it getting back to parents [where I teach]. Some work friends know, but they also know not to spread it around. That doesn't stress me out that much. I can defend that part of my life if I need to – I just don't want the extra work.

'I have friends outside of work who are also poly and they're a good support network. I'm very glad they exist. I'm also in some online communities which I love.'

The question that Dr Martin hears the MOST when it comes to women thinking about alternatives to monogamy? *'Am I normal?'*

Yes, we're back to the question that sits at the heart of so much of what we've been talking about in this book.

'When you look comprehensively and comparatively at the data from primatology, anthropology, sex research, medicine – what you see is that the range of "normal" is extremely wide,' says Dr Martin.

'If you are a woman who is struggling with monogamy, you are very normal indeed. There is nothing wrong with you. And that's a message I really want women to internalise. If you enjoy monogamy, that's normal too. We've evolved as very flexible, social and sexual strategists. There are many relationship styles and containers that can serve us for a while.

'But I would tell women one last thing, which is that being truly sexually excited about someone over and over and over again for years and years on end does *not* conform to any known scientific model we have about how we habituate to a stimulus over time and how we desensitise to excitement over time.

'So if you're a woman and you are bored and you are having service sex and you are tempted – you are NORMAL. Or if you are a woman who says monogamy is really not for me, there is nothing wrong with you.'

Claudia married young, and after her divorce, she went into her second marriage with the explicit intention of never again trying to be monogamous. She met her secondary partner two years ago. 'It's intoxicating! There are no drugs that could substitute for having this man There's an element of taboo about it as well because I live with my older partner and the big age difference with my younger guy is a taboo.

'At certain times I am definitely having more sex than most people. I get that variety as well. But that's not what it's all about. I think it's about knowing that you have someone who has that commitment to you. A marriage certificate doesn't stop people from leaving you or cheating.

'You need to make sure you're both onboard because there is a bit of a trope that the husband thinks he'll open up the relationship and get ALL THIS SEX, and in reality it's his wife who's getting all the sex and he's at home looking after the kids.'

According to Dr Martin, almost a third of married women who are refusing monogamy describe their relationships as happy or very happy. That's right – an existing happy relationship is key to having a successful open relationship.

'Sometimes I get couples coming to see me and they may have sexual problems or other relationship problems and they think by opening up the relationship, that might solve a lot. But that is definitely the wrong reason to go into it,' says Spierings.

'Polyamory is successful when people feel they have a really good, solid primary relationship. Then they go into these secondary relationships, whether that's openly shared with one another, or whether one partner does their own thing.

'I often say to people to maybe consider a sacred element that's just for the primary couple. So that might be kissing. Let's agree that's just for us. You don't do that with anybody else, or it might be a special restaurant that you share.

'There is often a very strong trust and commitment level in terms of the primary relationship. That's quite beautiful to see.'

'Every relationship is different. And I think it would be good if we could all have a better understanding of that. At the end of the day, it's about the couple or the individuals involved. If they're happy? Good on them. That contract only concerns them. So if it's agreed to and consented to by those individuals, it can really work.'

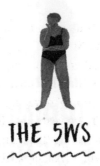

THE 5WS

Desiree Spierings says if you are thinking about opening up your relationship, you'll need to really think through the details, and the more detail the better. The 5Ws can be a good way to start thinking and talking to your partner about poly.

1. **Why** you are doing this? Is it purely about sex? Is it about wanting a deeper emotional connection to other people? Is it that your relationship isn't working for you? The answers will help you to decide on the kind of relationships you want to pursue.

2. **Who** are you allowed to see in this relationship? Is it only strangers? Is it people you know? What about colleagues or friends? Can you only see people who live a long way from your primary relationship? Also, who's allowed to know about what's happening in your relationship? Is it an open thing that you are going to tell your friends and family about? Or is it just between the two of you?

3. **What** are the types of things you are able to do with new partners? Can you go on dates? Can you go on long-stay holidays? Can you just hang out and go to the supermarket? What types of sexual activities are you able to do?

4. **When** can you see other people? Only during certain times or days? How much time can you spend with them?

5. **Where** are you able to spend time with other partners? Are you able to go out in public? Will you go to your favourite places? Can they come to your house?

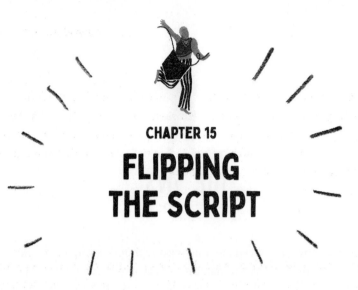

CHAPTER 15
FLIPPING THE SCRIPT

O ver the years, an unofficial community has grown around the podcast. These cool, kind, smart and brave humans get in touch to tell us how the stories we share give them knowledge and courage, help them feel less alone and ashamed, and open their minds about their own experiences and those of others. It's the best thing about working on *Ladies, We Need To Talk*.

But there are two episodes in particular that have drawn loads of honest and heartfelt responses. These episodes were about women who rejected two major tranches of what society considers intrinsic to womanhood: MARRIAGE and MOTHERHOOD.

After the episodes dropped, many in our community reached out to tell us that, yes, there are two sides to this story.

Ladies team, thanks for today's episode. I've been single going on eight years, and I fucking love it. I am the happiest person I know. I'm smart. Interesting. Well travelled. Funny. But do you know what everyone wants to know about? Am I seeing someone? For fuck's sake, can we talk about something else? – **KATE**

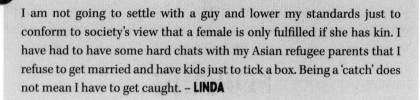

I am not going to settle with a guy and lower my standards just to conform to society's view that a female is only fulfilled if she has kin. I have had to have some hard chats with my Asian refugee parents that I refuse to get married and have kids just to tick a box. Being a 'catch' does not mean I have to get caught. – **LINDA**

Thank you for the latest episode about being childfree by choice. I knew I didn't want my own kids by the time I was 16. I spent a few years thinking maybe I'll adopt or foster. By the time I was 22 I realised adoption or fostering weren't for me. I'm 28 now and hugely on board with being childfree. Thank you for validating my decision, making me feel OK about it and being a voice against the huge chorus of 'you'll change your mind', 'you will feel differently when you have your own' and 'children are the best thing ever'. – **RHIANNON**

Here's the life plan as most of our parents see it: You're born, you grow up, you get a job, you get married, you have a family, you watch your kids grow up and maybe live a version of that get-married-have-kids script themselves, and THEN YOU DIE! It's a narrative that leaves little room for anything else.

And while in recent decades some of the details have changed and improved, that key bit of script about marrying or partnering and having a baby? It hasn't. We're still expected to find a partner and start a family.

For some, being single or not having children aren't active choices, and a lot of the storytelling on the podcast has centred around infertility and last-shot pregnancy. Sometimes life delivers surprises we didn't ask for or want. Those experiences can be devastating and they can come with an all-consuming grief. It is no small thing and we acknowledge your experience. If this is you, please take care choosing whether to read on, as some of the following material may trigger uncomfortable feelings or memories.

In this chapter we are talking about the women who ACTIVELY CHOOSE to be single or to not have children, or both. The women who have chosen to deviate from the story that has been written for us.

Ladies, we need to talk about FLIPPING THE SCRIPT.

✳ ✳ ✳

'As a woman, there's this kind of cultural ideal that's fairly cross-cultural that you're supposed to want to nurture and care,' says Dr Zoë Krupka, a feminist psychotherapist, researcher and lecturer at the Cairnmillar Institute in Melbourne. 'When you say, "I don't want to do that," it's like you're not a real woman or not a grown-up woman.'

Female identity is so interwoven with the idea of caring for others, especially partners and family, that any word used to describe an experience outside of this is imbued with negativity: spinster, lonely, neglectful, barren, childless, desolate, unfruitful, immature ...

There's also a belief that women who are single or childfree are 'selfish'. But social scientist Dr Bella DePaulo says when you look at the research, women in these categories are among those who contribute MOST to our society through acts of service and volunteering.

'A great study of Australian women, 10,000 Australian women, 70 and older, compared the ones who were single, had always been single and have no kids, to every other variety: married with children; married without children; previously married, with children, without, so on. It's the lifelong single women with no kids who volunteer the most.

'It's the single people who are giving more when somebody needs something from the little things in everyday life, like a ride somewhere, or help with an errand or yard work. Whatever it is, single people are consistently there more often than married people.'

I'm a single person on the autism spectrum. It's not depressing to me that I'm single. I'm pretty happy, because I've achieved a lot. I have explored relationships before, but short-term ones, and dating and stuff. But as much as I enjoy experiencing that, I feel as though I can accomplish a lot more on my own. When I think about the future, I think about how I can have an impact, rather than what me and my partner can do. – **CARLA**

'There was a study that followed people who have been single all their lives and married people over a course of five years,' says Dr DePaulo. 'And they found that over that five-year period, people who stayed single experienced more personal growth.'

Take a moment to think about how this statement sits alongside the stories of the single women we see play out on our screens or in the pages of our books. These fictional women are always ... *incomplete*.

Sex and the City, a show literally about being a single woman, sold out its own premise and made the main character marry a thoroughly shitty man in the end. Beyoncé's hit song 'Single Ladies' doesn't celebrate single ladies so much as urge them to move on to another man because the last one didn't offer marriage. And has there been a more damning depiction of singledom than Cinderella's 'ugly stepsisters'?

Can society imagine that someone who's single might be happy about it? We assume every single person wishes for a different life, that every 'happily ever after' comes with a plus one.

In reality, many of the single women we spoke to feel ... fine. They're happy! They're not waiting for anything! They value having time and brain space to think about what is meaningful for them, and then putting in place a plan to achieve those things. Are they totally happy, all the time? Nope. But are you?

Dr DePaulo has written a book called *Singled Out* and she is very familiar with the narratives that dominate how we think about single women. 'People think if you're single, you're miserable and you're lonely, and you don't have a life, and you have nothing to do but play. Then there's the other belief that if you're single, what you want more than anything else in the world is to become coupled.

'It turns out that just about all of these stereotypes about single people that are so widely shared are either grossly exaggerated or just plain wrong.'

Research across the human life span shows **our happiness has less to do with our relationship status and more to do with our own personal happiness set point**.

'The most rigorous studies are showing that when people get married, they don't get any healthier at all. And happiness? The very best possibility, and this doesn't happen in all of the studies, is that when people first get married, they get a little blip of happiness, like they're on their honeymoon and they just have this big party ... and it's all so exciting. But then when you follow them the next year, the year after that, their happiness starts to slip. It goes back to where they're just as happy or as unhappy as they were when they were single,' says Dr DePaulo.

Jane Mathews is an author and marketing consultant who has written a book called *The Art of Living Alone and Loving It*. 'There are more people living alone in Australia than there ever have been,' she says. 'There's about two million people.'

In her late 50s, and a decade from her divorce, Jane says she sees herself being single forever. 'I don't see myself ever getting together with anyone. Not a long-term relationship.'

Jane says this for two reasons: because finding a decent partner close to her age who's able 'to read without moving his lips' is like finding 'unicorn tears'; and because the longer she's alone, the more self-sufficient she becomes.

When you're single because of a relationship breakdown in later life, the adjustment can be tricky for your peer group. It comes down to those expectations again. When your story is outside of the conventional script, it confuses people.

'When I got divorced, probably about half of my friends, I would say, didn't invite me to anything ever again,' says Jane. 'I didn't realise that being married was part of the cost of entry into that social circle.

'There are times when it's not loneliness, it's not Christmas Day, it's not holidays by myself … it's getting the top off a fucking jar in the evening when I'm by myself! I have to go to my next-door neighbour and say, "Can you take the top off?" Yeah, that's really awful.'

Jane's approach to being single is similar to how we're encouraged to think about relationships – you need to put in consistent work and effort.

'It starts by actually liking yourself and being happy in yourself. If you don't like what you see when you look in the mirror – not necessarily physically – but you're going to spend all this time by yourself, so you have to like it. And if you do, then you can kill it at being single. But if you're not happy by yourself, then you'll never be happy. And I enjoy my own company.

'Suze Orman, this finance woman in America, said that she liked herself so much, she'd date herself. She had a crush on herself. I can't imagine myself ever saying anything like that. But I quite admire her chutzpah, because she likes being with herself.'

So happiness isn't connected to whether or not we're partnered. But this truth hasn't filtered through to popular perception.

Jane says, 'The perception of a single person is someone who feels that they are missing out … That they're one of society's outliers, that they will definitely be eaten by the cat when they fall down the stairs, and that they won't leave as big a mark on the world. The reality is that I intend to leave a very big mark on the world and I am content and I don't yearn for someone to complete me.'

'The perception is that I'm lonely and I'm going to die alone,' says Andy, who's in her late 40s and has been single for more than 15 years. 'It is also that I'm footloose and fancy free. The reality is that I am really connected to a lot of people and I have a lot of love in my life and a lot of richness. And I just refuse to just take up one space and buy a unit. I want a big backyard and a garden and just this richness.'

✳ ✳ ✳

At best, women who have flipped the script on having a partner are misunderstood. At worst, they're pitied. But what about the women – with or without a partner – who bluntly refuse to have kids?

Dr Krupka defines 'childfree by choice' as a woman making a conscious decision that she doesn't want to have her own children.

'Childfree by choice doesn't mean she doesn't want to co-parent or step-parent or help her friends out with their kids or be an aunty, but she's made a conscious decision that's not based on infertility or chance or circumstances beyond her control.'

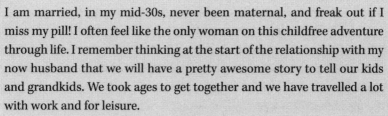

I am married, in my mid-30s, never been maternal, and freak out if I miss my pill! I often feel like the only woman on this childfree adventure through life. I remember thinking at the start of the relationship with my now husband that we will have a pretty awesome story to tell our kids and grandkids. We took ages to get together and we have travelled a lot with work and for leisure.

But as time went by and questions started coming about when we would have kids, we came to the conclusion that us contributing to the world's population was not a priority. We both have nieces and nephews to play with and although people say I will get clucky, I cringe. – **NADIA**

It's a fascinating paradox. As modern feminists we believe profoundly in a woman's right to choose what happens to her body – particularly around reproduction. But for some reason there's a weird blind spot. Yes, we think she has the right to choose – so long as she *eventually* chooses to have children! 'Don't wait too long!' We've heard it a thousand times, maybe even said it ourselves? The script around the 'glorious fulfilment' that comes with child rearing can sometimes override our understanding that the sacred right to choose includes the right to choose not to have kids EVER.

> People always think I need a reason or need to justify my decision to not have my own kids. I am a 31-year-old stepmother to a 20-year-old boy and a 15-year-old girl (I was 26 when my stepson came to live with us full time). Is that why I don't want kids? No. I work in advertising, not the easiest career to have as a mother or be a female in – full stop. Is that my reason? No.
>
> My partner would have a baby if I wanted to. My reasons are completely my own, and sometimes I can't even explain it – I just know that I don't want my own kids. I say to people, if a child needed fostering, or there was a baby in need, I would take them in and raise them. The preconception that I am not maternal or don't like kids is completely untrue. I love caring for people and animals, love my nephews, my friends' children, but my rescue dogs are also my life (crazy dog lady).
>
> I've heard 'You should be a mother' (this was last week when I was holding a stranger's baby at a work video shoot) or 'All women are meant to be mothers' or 'You'd be a great mum, you need to have kids', and my absolute favourite – 'Well, not everyone is meant for motherhood'. That one annoys me most because maybe I am meant for motherhood. I would be a fucking awesome mum, but I STILL choose not to have my own kids. What is so hard to get across to the judgemental people (my family included) is that I know I would be a great mum, but the choice is still mine. – **BEC**

People's reasons for choosing not to have children are complex.

One big one is the unrelenting expectations that our society places on mothers. 'It's to all of that "perfect mother" ideal that a lot of women are going, "I'm not interested,"' says Dr Krupka. 'I think you can understand that if you are a mother, because you have an idea about what that perfectionism actually feels like.

'They're seeing that around them and going, "That's not what I want. I don't want to have to meet that terrible standard."'

A 2019 study from The Australian Conservation Foundation and 1 Million Women found that some women might choose not to have children because of concerns about overpopulation and climate change. A 2013 Deakin University study found that some women might not feel a maternal instinct, or perhaps have health concerns or a desire for independence and freedom.

Truth is that many women have several reasons for making their choice.

Carly Findlay is an author and activist, who was born with a chronic skin condition called ichthyosis. She's very clear that she doesn't want kids, but gets frustrated by the assumptions people make as to why she's made her choice.

'People think that disabled people are not sexual, or not maternal. When I was growing up, the kids at school told me I'd never have sex. They assumed that my appearance and skin was too much of a deterrent. When I met Adam I hadn't dated much before really, and people were genuinely happy for me but would ask my mum (not me), "Does he have ichthyosis too?" – pointing to their faces.

'About four days after I got married, I went to a women in leadership event as a guest speaker. Five women asked, "So when are the babies coming?" – at a leadership conference!'

Carly also has to deal with the assumption that she'll pass on her skin condition to her offspring. 'When a baby is born with a disability it's seen as a tragedy. So the idea that I might have a baby and pass it on is seen as irresponsible! A polite reminder that that is my life story!

'Extended family have advised me against having children because I would be a burden on my husband! For me, when it comes from strangers, it's hard, but when it comes from someone who's close to you, it's worse.

'My condition is severe and very rare. Most parents [with ichthyosis] would have a one in four chance of having a child with this condition. People imply you should have a termination or shouldn't have a child at all or you should do embryo selection. It's very hard when people weigh in. They think that a child being born like me would be the WORST thing that could happen! It's projection of their own biases around what disability is – it's ableism.'

Journalist and commentator Tory Shepherd decided to tackle the stigma that childfree women face in her book *On Freedom*, which studies the impacts of our ability to actively choose motherhood.

Tory has known she didn't want kids since high school. It was common knowledge among her friends. Still she was surprised that people were making assumptions about her character based on her decision not to have kids. 'I was going to a series of baby showers and running into people who know me and know that I don't want kids. They assumed that I hate kids. I got the "Why are you at your friend's baby shower, you don't even like kids?"

'So then I had this epiphany: "Oh, that's the stigma – that I am an unnatural witchy person."'

In Tory's book, she looks at the narratives around women who don't have kids, including comments made in the public domain by men in very powerful positions.

Like the 2016 speech that Turkish President Recep Tayyip Erdoğan gave to a *women's democracy association conference,* where he said that women's lives were incomplete if they didn't have children. (He urged women to have at least three kids and said 'rejecting motherhood means giving up on humanity'.)

Then there was the time our first female prime minister, Julia Gillard, was called 'deliberately barren' by an old male senator, who argued she couldn't make decisions about family policy because she couldn't understand how families work – without her own kids.

Ex-politician Emma Husar talks about the 'Julia effect'.

'So when Julia Gillard was our first female prime minister, I think we saw the worst of society's diatribe and gender inequality and disrespect. The vitriol that she was subjected to – you couldn't help but feel such a massive degree of empathy for how much harder her job was simply because she was a woman and she was judged not on what was coming out of her mouth or the policies that she brought to us, but how she's decided to remain childless. She's not married.

'Maybe people weren't talking about that invisible judgement openly but I certainly felt the Julia effect.'

'All of it's utter tosh, but it does kind of bang away in the background,' says Tory. 'I don't know how much other women feel that "if you don't use your womb you're not really a woman". I think as much as you can consciously reject those assumptions, it's really hard to be sure that none of it is squirming its way into the backdrop of your mind.'

Another argument that childfree women often face is that kids are your tilt at immortality. It's not surprising – humans have a long track record of doing crazy things so they can live forever. 'It's sort of a fantasy, really – "I'm gonna live on because my kids will remember me and their kids will remember me,"' says Dr Krupka. 'Really, that's not going to matter to you because *you'll be dead.'*

Then there's the suggestion that you will die sad and alone with no-one to look after you. Tory reckons you should be able to hire someone to look after you with all the money you've saved from not having a kid. And a LOT of people have got in touch to point out how gross it is to put the burden of looking after you in old age on your offspring – a little bit like breeding your own help.

Caroline has been married for more than 20 years and says she has never felt maternal and her husband didn't have strong feelings either way. Before they married, the pair made their decision not to have kids and, despite exhortations to change their minds, it's a decision they've never regretted. They travel. They have plenty of pets and horses. They hang out with friends and family, including other people's kids.

Caroline still finds that people assume she has kids. 'You'll meet someone, say in a work environment or a new environment, and they'll say, "So how old are your kids?" And I just say, "I don't have any." Then there's this stunned silence and some other kind of comment, "Ah, so that's how you get to go on holidays."

'I don't think my husband has the same conversations that I've had over the years. I remember an older friend of mine, we'd go for our little horse rides in the bush and she was so worried that I'd made this decision and it really concerned her. I had to convince her I'd be fine. I remember she said, "You should have them because you might regret it when you're older." And I said, "Look, I'd be selfish if I had them because I might regret it."'

Dr Krupka says the 'you'll regret it' argument is often put forward for why women should have kids, but we talk a lot less about the women who did have kids and then regretted it.

'These aren't easy choices. You can't make them perfectly. We all do the best that we can in terms of the choices that we're able to make. Absolutely, there will be some who regret not having children. But there isn't really a significant amount when you're looking at women who've made that active choice, which is really interesting. Far fewer than those that regret having children.'

Hang on. Did you catch that? We're going to repeat it in case you missed it. Based on her clinical work with women and the research she's seen, Dr Krupka says **more women regret choosing to have children than regret choosing not to have children**.

Caroline also had friends who believed in her. 'My close girlfriends have always been really supportive and probably know that it's absolutely the right decision. They've always said it would be absolutely hilarious if I did get pregnant.

'One of my close girlfriends has said, "I love that I have a friend who doesn't have children, because it's really good to talk to you about stuff. You look at it from an outsider's point of view, and you often come out with quite a different perspective on things."'

Caroline's had the support of her family as well. Her mother even told Caroline and her sister that if she could have her time again she probably would've chosen to be childfree as well. 'Mum was totally on board. My dad was fine with it as well. My husband's family struggled with it a little bit more, especially his mum. But she's grown after all these years. She's realised that we're both happy.'

When performer Jess Saras told her dad she wasn't going to have kids, she was surprised by how his response made her feel. 'He was like, "Oh, so I'm never going to be a grandfather." That kind of hit me. More than I expected. I was like, "Oh, shit. OK." To see that and see him being a little bit sad. That was the one time I felt guilty.'

Jess's decision surprised her family because mothering had been such a big part of her own mum's life, and Jess had grown up thinking it's what all women did. Until she got older and started to discover what was important to her and what she wanted to do with her life.

'I was in a relationship, my last long-term relationship, which was seven years ago, and it was like the "settle" trial for me. It meant moving to his place of work and being the caretaker. If we were still together, it would have led to children and his career advancement, and not mine. For the last 10 months of that relationship, I was miserable, and then totally hit rock bottom, and did all of this soul searching and ... kind of gradually built myself back up. I really came to that clarity of what was right for me, what I wanted to do with my life. And kids were just not in the picture.'

Her family and friends have supported her decision. 'They respect my choice as well. The criticism has come more from an outside perspective. So people that are not really that close to me, they're just like, "You have to settle down one day." And I say, "But *why* do I have to? Explain to me why I have to. I don't want to. I'm totally happy being by myself."'

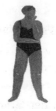

HOW TO BE A BETTER ALLY TO YOUR SCRIPT-FLIPPING MATES

Respect your friends' decision. If your friend came out as gay, you wouldn't try to talk them out of it. You would accept what they said, not assume you know better. Because you don't know what is inside their heart better than they do, no matter how much you love them, right? Whether it's not having children, not partnering, going poly or any other decision they make – true friendships THRIVE on acceptance.

What's the lingo? If they're a close friend, ask or follow their lead. 'Childless' might not be your friends' preferred way to put it; some people like 'childfree'. Others might not want to be defined by their relationship status; as Sarah told us, 'I don't identify as single. I identify as Sarah.'

Childfree doesn't mean they don't like kids. There are definitely some people who don't like kids. But they're often parents! Being childfree and disliking children don't automatically go together.

Having children is a personal decision. It isn't anyone's business who is or isn't having children. Don't ask unless you're very close. And if you're not? Allow them to volunteer what information they want to volunteer.

'You might regret it' is a dumb thing to say. You might regret that butterfly tattoo you got on your lower back in Byron Bay but your friend didn't try to talk you out of that, did she? Yes, they've thought it through. No, really, they've thought it through.

'Have you met anyone?' and 'Are you seeing someone?' are also dumb things to say. Those are annoying questions. If that's the best you can come up with for a conversation starter? Try harder. If they HAVE met someone and they want to share it? They'll definitely tell you.

Set-ups need to be thought through. Every unpartnered person has been set up with someone who is completely inappropriate because a well-meaning friend has thought, 'They're single and my good friend is single, I'll set them up!' It's not enough that two people have singledom in common and nothing else. Look for common ground before you start playing Cupid.

Single people don't need your pity. The only thing missing from the life of a person choosing to be single is the approval of broader society. Your pity isn't helping, isn't needed, and is actually kind of arrogant. 'I wish people would believe me when I say I'm not masking a deep sadness that I haven't met someone. I am genuinely very happy on my own,' says Courtney.

Consider their point of view. They've helped every other person celebrate weddings. Engagements. Births and birthdays. Maybe they want to be celebrated? Do they need a big moment of recognition? And if everyone else gets to bring a plus one, maybe they want to as well?

They don't need to be in a couple to hang out with you. Single people are used to being single. They're not going to be weirded out if they're asked to sit at a table with three other couples. Try it out. Single people also don't have that default 'mate' to hang out with in their spare time so are often bang up for doing fun stuff.

P.S. Single people DON'T WANT TO BE PART OF YOUR THREESOME. Or maybe they do? Who are we to say? But definitely help a sister out by opening a jar for her when she asks, OK? They put those jar lids on so goddamn tight.

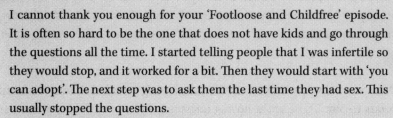

I cannot thank you enough for your 'Footloose and Childfree' episode. It is often so hard to be the one that does not have kids and go through the questions all the time. I started telling people that I was infertile so they would stop, and it worked for a bit. Then they would start with 'you can adopt'. The next step was to ask them the last time they had sex. This usually stopped the questions.

Finally having someone explain that we are not selfish, heartless women is wonderful! I feel like my husband and I have been able to do so much more for my family because we do not have kids. We moved back to live with them to help them out due to health issues. I wish you could translate this into Spanish so I can send it to my mother-in-law and my husband's family. But I will take solace in the fact that the word is getting out there that we are just normal people. – **FRANCES**

Flipping the script requires courage because you don't get to look around you and see other people doing what you are doing.

Even though Tory has always known she didn't want kids, she was almost caught in the motherhood slipstream. It's hard to overestimate how powerful it can be – to finally feel like you're following the script that almost everyone you know has stuck to.

'I fell in love. I moved in with a guy. I got married. I thought it was all clear that we weren't going to reproduce, and then things kind of shifted. It got to a point where I thought, "Why don't we just try, because everyone tells me I'll be so happy if it happens." So we tried that for a while. But the feeling I got every time I got my period, I'd never been so frickin' happy to see that little bastard in my life. That made me know that doing this to keep everyone happy was probably not the correct path.'

Eventually it got to the point where it became clear that she and her former husband weren't going to agree. 'The word "deal-breaker" was bandied around. It's never as simple as that, but that was the deal-breaker in my marriage in the end.'

Jess has some pretty compelling reasons for why she doesn't want to have kids – high up on her list is climate change. 'It really worries me. What kind of world, if I do have a child, am I going to raise it in? What problems are we passing on to them? It's really tough. It's even harder to hear my parents and other older family members that are like, "Well, I'll be gone. It's not my problem." If I have your grandchildren, it's their problem, so how is it not your problem now?'

If I say I don't have kids, the default reaction is pity! I can see their faces – they don't want to say the wrong thing but they're scrolling through the options: *is she infertile, a dating loser* … They offer pity, not congratulations! On the few occasions I have actually discussed it with people, they say, 'Yeah, but who's gonna look after you in old age?' I don't think there's enough resources for all of us to have children. Some of us are going to have to choose not to have babies for environmental reasons. – **JULIE**

Carly Findlay also has many reasons for choosing not to have kids. 'I don't have a child because I really like my freedom and I don't like poo. I *really* don't like poo! Also – it's expensive! I want my weekends and I want to spend money on things that matter to me.

'When I'm old I want to be wearing really bright clothes and surrounding myself with good friends, reading and writing and still being loud. I will measure my success by how confident I've made other people. Making them confident to tell their story, wear what they want, or not hide their skin condition. That will be the measure of a good life.'

Flipping the script is what we all do when we refuse to be shamed by things that traditionally have been used to squash us and mortify us. Whether we shamelessly walk our fat bodies down the beach, unapologetically seek support for our leaking, fanny-farting bodies, love our vaginas and the pleasure our clits bring – it's all glorious and messy and part of a great un-learning. And unlearning shame and taboo is what *Ladies, We Need To Talk* has been about from the start.

WHAT PEOPLE WANT YOU TO KNOW

Yumi asked on social media: 'If you're single by choice, and/or childless by choice – what do you wish you could tell your friends and family?' The messages came in – it wasn't so much a deluge of messages as an avalanche. Here's a sample, using the posters' social media handles.

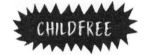

Please stop telling me that I should have children because I'm so good with kids. – **LA.TESTA.ROSSA**

A. It's definitely, 100% not a phase. B. Yes, I know my partner and I would have 'really cute kids'. C. I have a long history of trauma and mental illness. This was as a result of being raised by parents with – you guessed it – significant trauma and mental health issues themselves. I wanted to break the chain of what is like a curse in my family, and I am so glad that this was my choice. – **TESQUILAX80**

So many women before me fought so hard to give me this luxury. I intend to fulfil that to the fullest. – **LINDA**

I wish other people, primarily other women TBH, would know that it's actually fucking rude to enquire as to why a woman hasn't had kids, what their intentions are around having kids, etc. It's 10/10 none of anyone else's goddamn business so please for the love of dog stop asking! – **PIPONABIKE**

When I say I'll babysit your kids, I mean it! I've chosen not to have a kid in my life 365 days a year ... but a few days a year is wonderful. – **JULIALENTON**

Please don't say, 'Oh, that's OK,' or try to reassure: we know it's OK. Also, I'm allowed to be tired. – **DOING.THERAPY**

I was accidentally pregnant once but felt huge relief when I miscarried. The miscarriage taught me to know for sure that I don't want kids. – **ANIKELLEY83**

I'd like society to be more accepting of women like me, who put their child into foster care – I don't fit in anywhere. – **NELLIEKBOLLINGMOORE**

I came to the decision to be childfree after a lifetime of default social programming that I would be a mum and I would definitely want to be one. From our births, so much of our life, decisions and the way society treats us is based on this assumption. Imagine instead what life would look like and what opportunities we may explore if the reverse were true – and being a mum was something we came to later in life, due to a deep desire to have them instead? – **SENSEANDSMASHABILITY**

I used to get frustrated with 'you'll change your mind' and the 'you have no idea' comment about parenting. I do have an idea and that's why I don't want to do it! Talk to me about literally anything other than dating apps and freezing my eggs! – **JESSWATUCKABEES**

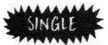

SINGLE

Celebrate my milestones, even though they are different to yours. – **LEILANIMASON**

I have been lonelier in past relationships. – **SLOWDOWNANDGROW**

I will never put myself in a situation where either myself or my child can be hurt by someone who lives in my house. I have friends and I love my life. I can find joy without needing a partner. – **TONI_ALTSWAGGER**

I'm learning to love myself before I can even try to love another. – **BREECARDWELL**

I wish I had just told people that I was 40 sooner so they could leave me the fuck alone. – **JEANETTEMASSIE**

Please stop treating me as though I haven't reached happiness, and won't until I am in a relationship. Please accept the journey I am on. Please support my journey in falling in love with myself. – **STRICTLY_DECAF**

I am content. – **COURTNEYACT**

People I meet for the first time think we were put here to pair up and procreate. – **TASHARA_ROBERTS**

I am not 'too picky'. – **NUT_MEG1828**

Stop saying I'll find someone when I least expect it. I have no interest in being romantically connected to anyone. – **SARAHMPHASER**

You need to be strong and confident to do things on your own but it is so worth it. – **EARTHTOKEZZA**

It's hard for a lot of people to understand that the prospect of a relationship can be really unappealing to some people. – **YVIE_JONES**

Don't tell me that one day I'll find someone else and live YOUR version of a fairy tale. Please don't tell me I'll change my mind. Perhaps I'm happy now. – **MARYANNEATALLA**

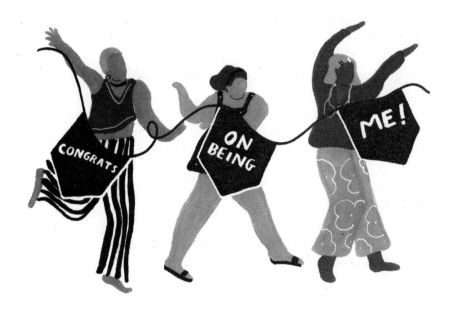

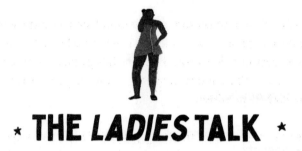

★ THE *LADIES* TALK ★

L adies, we need to say thank you. Thank you for reading, and thank you for being part of *Ladies, We Need To Talk*. We did not anticipate this incredible outcome when we gently shoved those first few seeds of an idea into the ground. But look! The forest is here, and it's cool and calm and there's space for everyone.

Claudine came up with the idea for the podcast, assembled an amazing crew, steered the *Ladies* ship out of the harbour in season one, and wrote this book. Yumi gets to voice the episodes, conduct the interviews and co-wrote this book. But besides us two, there is a team of hard-working women working behind the scenes. Because the podcast has been running for more than five years, people come and go. But whether they were onboard for a single season or the whole time, all the ladies involved have had a BLAST making the show. Naturally, they have something to say about the experience.

So in the spirit of closing the loop in this book, we'd like to end with some words from them.

★

I remember getting a call from Claudine telling me a pilot season of *Ladies, We Need To Talk* was happening and thinking *YES!* Not because I was being asked to join the team, but because this show was finally going to exist. A space unapologetically for women, by women, about women.

We started off by listing all the things in our lives we felt were not being properly talked about in the media, or in some cases not being talked about at all. Which ultimately led to conversations about the nuances of the female and non-binary experience and the tricky parts of feminism. And finally to some very real conversations with our guests, who so generously shared their stories and floored me with their vulnerability and integrity.

By the end of the first season, emails from listeners were starting to roll in and the beginning of a community was in the making. A community who wanted to be part of a conversation about things that aren't always easy to talk about, but are talked about anyway, in a way that was real and messy and true. – **JESS BINETH, producer**

★

I remember the night before the first episode of *Ladies* was ever released. I was racked with nerves and excitement and checked the podcast app at least every half hour until about 5 am when the little pink tile finally appeared – we were live!

It's been a total joy to watch *Ladies* go from strength to strength, and to see conversations that felt taboo just four years ago become increasingly mainstream. What I love most about the show is the many interesting, funny, and honest discussions it's sparked, and the wonderful community it's created. – **OLIVIA WILLIS, producer**

★

Being a part of the *Ladies* team has honestly been such a joy in my life. It's quite possibly been the highlight of my 34-year career. I love that I'm entrusted with shaping the audio picture for each episode and that I'm given the autonomy to be creative (and to make fart noises from time to time). It's nourishing for the soul.

Working from home during the pandemic has meant my family gets to see the range of emotions I'm feeling as I'm editing. They watch me go from laughter, to tears, to gasping, often all in the space of the same episode. And I've learnt so much from making the series – often I'll be furiously googling as I'm listening ... *what does a clitoris actually look like?* – **ANN-MARIE DEBETTENCOR, sound engineer**

★

Every so often (and actually it's *not* very often in the entertainment biz), you get to work on a show where all the ingredients come together in just the right way, at exactly the right time. *Ladies, We Need To Talk* is one of those shows. It quickly racked up record downloads, but more than that, we built a community of women around it. They started sharing stories they'd never told anyone – about their odd vaginas, weird smells, why they hated being a mother, how much they tried to avoid sex/have way more sex.

Everyone is changed in some way by working on *Ladies*. There's been so much fun, some tears, some odd looks from colleagues, and many snort-

laughs at the funnier things our bodies do. But best of all? I once got to shout across a busy newsroom: 'Team, we are not doing "Anal Sex" until we've done "Masturbation". And please bring forward "Porn" so it's before "Libido".'
– **KELLIE RIORDAN**, commissioning editor

★

I'm not really a small talk kind of person. It's big talk that's interesting. Honest, vulnerable, dirty, shocking and deep talk. That's where the good stuff is.

When we were developing a new season of *Ladies*, I remember sitting in an office in Sydney, surrounded by women I had never worked with before. Perhaps some polite small talk to begin? Not likely. We began, not by talking about the weather or whether to cut a fringe, but by telling each other a secret that we hadn't told anyone before. Big talk. Big yes. It was like drunk girl conversations in the bathrooms at a nightclub, only it was daytime, it was the workplace, and there was no alcohol in sight. Just women sharing secrets. Backing each other. Arguing. Laughing. Crying. Sharing the ugly and the beautiful.

That's why this show is so important, so valuable and so loved. It gets deep, unashamedly so. And it's the podcast equivalent of an entire bathroom stall of women nodding, rubbing your back, wiping away your tears and cheering you on. – **MONIQUE BOWLEY**, executive producer

★

There are very few jobs where you are likely to find yourself recording your own internal vaginal exam for the radio. But that's exactly what happened while I was working on *Ladies, We Need To Talk*. It was pretty odd and a little awkward, but I was nowhere near as brave as so many of the ladies who spoke to us for the show. It never ceased to amaze me how many women were willing to share stories they had never told before, in the hope that it might help someone else. We asked if they wanted to remain anonymous, but often they would tell us they'd be happy to use their real names because, in telling their stories, they realised they were proud of those experiences and how they had shaped their lives. – **MADELEINE GENNER**, supervising producer

★

I cherish so much of my time on *Ladies*. My feminism evolved so much; I became more intersectional in my lens. Yumi turned me into a mad runner (and probably a better cook). As a result of the 'Secret Life of Hormones' episode, I learnt I was hormonally sensitive and pushed hard to get myself an answer. I'm now on a contraception that makes me feel level, normal and cool!

I also realised through the experience of working on the show that I wanted to become a clinical psychologist, and I'm now well on my way.

But what I'll cherish most are the mates we became making this cool thing for the world. Female friendship – it's sacred! And it's what'll get you through.
– **CASSANDRA STEETH**, producer and supervising producer

Ladies is the best show I work on – and not just because the women I work with rock my world. Working on it has changed me. I know more about my body than I ever did. I now heartily embrace the use of the words vulva and discharge. I can put a term to things I never really had words to describe or explain, like the mental load and coercive control. I see the patriarchy and its evil tentacles (testicles?!) everywhere. Sure, it makes me bloody tiresome at parties when I go on and on about how it's the patriarchy's fault (it is BTW) and that we should band together and smash it, but this show has changed my view on the world, my place in it, my white privilege and the way I approach my life as a woman. In telling women's stories and talking about the universal issues we face as women, we're saying 'we see you', and that's powerful.
– **JUSTINE KELLY**, executive producer

Working on the podcast reminded me how change can happen when we share our stories, especially ones we're told are taboo or shameful. After hearing women telling their stories in their own words (or maybe in the form of a kooky debate about pubic hair removal between Pubis Maximus and Team Dolphin), hopefully we can all feel less weird, less ashamed, more empathic and more 'ourselves'. And revel in how freaking hilarious and excellent women can be. Thank you to all the women whose stories keep chipping away at the patriarchy to bring about safety and justice and a better world for everybody.
– **JANE CURTIS**, producer

We're getting ready to record an interview for *Ladies* in Studio 252. Tamar is producing today and she's talking to Yumi, who's going through her notes on the other side of the glass. Meanwhile, I get our guest on the line and check the levels. She's sounding good, so we hit record and settle in to hear her story.

I started working at the ABC too late to work on the legendary *Coming Out Show*, but I did listen to it, and loved it's daring and fearless airing of women's issues. *Ladies, We Need To Talk* has the same drive to delve into stories that matter to women, without apologising for confronting the tough issues.

Sometimes making the listener feel uncomfortable is the best way to tell a story, but it's vital to lighten up too. All the women working on *Ladies* are curious, smart, empathic and witty. They pick gritty topics, seek out fascinating guests and package up the stories with respect.

... Back in the studio, we're listening as the woman describes her traumatic birth experience. It's graphic and brave and powerful. And visceral – I realise that I've been simultaneously holding my breath and tensing my body as she speaks about the pain in hers. I'm hooked; it's going to be another must-listen episode. Thanks *Ladies*! – **JEN PARSONAGE, sound engineer**

★

Prior to working on *Ladies*, I used to listen obsessively on the train home from work – a decent commute that would allow me to chew through about three eps every arvo. I remember laughing out loud in public till a bit of pee came out, crying at the personal and heartbreaking stories that women would generously share, and I felt my blood boil as conversations around the orgasm gap and the mental load opened my eyes to the shit women deal with daily.

Starting work on a wildly successful, groundbreaking and taboo-smashing podcast in its fifth season is not an un-daunting thing ... Getting the call was equal parts *OMFG they want ME to make that awesome pod?* and *OMFG I have anxiety tummy*. As supervising producer, I help to shape the ideas, content and direction of the episodes, decide who might be interesting to hear from and make lots of often uncomfortable phone calls asking people to share their deepest, darkest secrets. The *Ladies* team is quite simply the most intelligent, sassy, supportive, open, caring and hilarious bunch of sheroes you could ever hope to be entangled with. – **ALEX LOLLBACK, supervising producer**

★

I was lucky enough to start working on *Ladies* in its fifth season, by which time it was already a well-oiled machine with a loyal following – including me. I remember waiting for new episodes to land and counting down the days between each season before Yumi would be back with sage advice, helping me learn things I never knew I needed to know.

Now that I'm part of the team, I'm constantly amazed at the things our guests share with us each episode; it's a real privilege to be entrusted with their stories, from the squishy to the sexy to the sad. The reason people feel safe to share the big stuff with us is because of the amazing, inclusive community that Yumi and all the producers have created. By sharing their stories, guests then pay it forward to other listeners who have their own stories validated or have their eyes opened to something new. I love seeing the way Yumi crafts the interviews and how she ties together our production with her brilliant writing, much of which makes me snort-laugh. I can't wait to see what we do next. – **TAMAR CRANSWICK, producer**

I was lucky enough to executive produce several episodes of *Ladies, We Need To Talk* – and I say lucky because it meant getting to hear all the parts we couldn't air. Highlights of the time include debating whether the term 'finger-banging' was widely used, workshopping episode titles like 'The Pelvic Flaw in All of Us' and having to justify whether a specific sex act deserved its own episode in a detailed brief. It was also the exact moment, after 35 years of life, that I learnt about hormones and the way they can both charge and drain us during our menstrual cycles. I want to blame my mum's reliance on the *What's Happening To Me* picture book for that lack of sex education but the truth is, there's just not enough information fed to young women about our sexual health. That's the beauty of *Ladies* for me. It's a place for the real-talk dissection of the things that matter to women – from mental loads, to sexual health, to friendship. – **LAURA MCAULIFFE, executive producer**

Ladies was my first ABC Audio Studios podcast. I was still very new to the ABC and at the time was undergoing training on more complex audio mixes. I was definitely thrown in the deep end and had to get over hearing blush-inducing stories over and over again. The thing about podcast mixing is you don't just hear the entire program once or twice or even three times! It takes many rounds to perfect a music cue, get a sound effect sitting just right or enhance an interview done over the phone. My squeamishness was short-lived, and I soon couldn't wait to see what the next mix had in store.

I was stoked to be able to work with so many talented women who bring the podcast to life, including highly respected and long-serving ABC sound engineer Judy Rapley. I've taken with me insight into the many issues concerning women today and have been blown away by how readily women have shared their stories to help and support each other. – **ISABELLA TROPIANO, sound engineer**

After a career spanning several decades, working on this series brought me full circle. I joined the ABC five years after the Australian Women's Broadcasting Cooperative was established. The first *Coming Out Show* went to air on ABC

Radio 2 (now Radio National) on International Women's Day 1975. It was a celebratory occasion – at last female voices and feminist perspectives had a public space. Women stepped out from behind typewriters to join seasoned producers, firmly grasping microphones and recorders, ready to fill the airwaves for that one hour a week. When I looked through the archives there are programs titled 'Love Gone Wrong', 'Warts and All – STDs that Kill' and 'Rape, the Neglected Crime'. From 1980, I mixed many of the unit's features until *Women Out Loud*, as it was renamed, was taken off air in 1998.

That leads me to 2018, when I joined the *Ladies, We Need To Talk* producers for the second series. It'd been a long time since women had a unique forum to tackle awkward topics, so I was delighted with the podcast's arrival and to be involved again. The show had already been 'bedded down' by a whip-sharp, creative and dedicated team, music composed by a talented ABC colleague. My job was to make the content sound as technically 'polished' as possible. And in collaboration with the supervising producer, I wove in themes, stings and sound effects adding texture to scripts and interviews. After such a long hiatus, it was enriching – thanks to the fabulous *Ladies* team – working with material specifically tailored for women.

Please ladies, keep on talking, LOUD! I'm still listening in my retirement!
– **JUDY RAPLEY**, technical producer

★

Making a book with *Ladies, We Need To Talk* was a dream project – important and joyful and collaborative, attempting to capture everything the podcast does so well in something you could hold in your hands and place in the hands of others. Making it also lined up with a time where things have felt HARD (see: 'Adding a Pandemic to the Equation' in chapter 7), but Claudine and Yumi and all the other clever, creative women involved in this book were the best people to spend that (virtual) time with. And I am really happy that I know so much more about discharge now. – **EMILY HART**, book commissioning editor

★

Ladies, We Need To Talk is the pep talk from our bestie that we all need when we're feeling ashamed or embarrassed or like we're the only ones in the world going through [insert 'secret women's business']. The more we speak up and share with our communities, the sooner we will realise that a diversity of experiences exist – and that we are not alone. It may also seem like the odds are stacked against us (patriarchy, anyone?), but if there's anything that *Ladies* has taught me, it's that we're stronger when we band together, when we possess knowledge and when we can fully appreciate all of the remarkable women in our lives. And, let's face it, it's probably the last time I'll be adding 'butt plug' to a style sheet! – **CAMHA PHAM, book editor**

I'm extremely grateful to have played a small part in the *Ladies, We Need To Talk* team. It is refreshing to see that there are books like these that take a very pragmatic, HUMAN approach to day-to-day issues. – **REG ABOS, book designer**

When I was approached to contribute to the *Ladies, We Need To Talk* book I was ecstatic! I love researching and writing about issues that affect women, especially our health. What I didn't expect was how much I would learn about myself and how this information would stick with me.

Speaking to women from my community of different ages and from different locations helped me realise that I wasn't alone in my experience. As an Aboriginal, Fijian/Indian woman, topics like periods, body image and anxiety are still very much taboo, but creating a space where we can openly and honestly discuss our lived experiences helped not only me but the women I spoke with to feel less alone. These topics also come with trauma, so for some (including myself) it was about reflecting on how that's shaped the way we feel, view and understand our body and ourselves; how it trickles into other areas of our life, like dating, motherhood and our career; and how we're learning to unapologetically embrace who we are and take this power back. – **TAHNEE JASH, book researcher**

★

The first time I realised that what I was calling the vagina is actually called the vulva was only a couple of years ago – and I learnt that from the *Ladies, We Need To Talk* podcast!

I loved working on this book because it took away some of the embarrassment of NOT knowing things – what a clitoris looks like, what an actual pelvic floor is! There was tonnes of coded language and shame around periods and sex in my family. I distinctly remember having to wrap my used pads in newspaper and chuck them in the outside wheelie bin because of the 'bad smell'. Reading other stories like mine made me feel less alone! I am so proud to have had the chance to not only be part of something so educational (and entertaining) but also to have had the extra bonus of learning along the way. – **GRACE LEE, book illustrator**

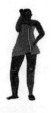

★ INDEX ★

★ ACKNOWLEDGEMENTS ★

We want to give a huge heartfelt thanks to all of the women who have shared their secrets, stories, expertise and insights, first on the podcast and now in these pages. Their words are the foundation stones on which the *Ladies, We Need To Talk* community is built.

Ladies, We Need To Talk would never have existed if it wasn't for season one's incredible production crew. Kellie Riordan, Jess Bineth and Olivia Willis – you will always have a very special place in our hearts for putting so much energy, love and bits of your soul into *Ladies*. A special shout-out to Marty Peralta – sound engineer, musician, the only man we let anywhere near the pod in season one, and the person responsible for creating the theme music with its distinctive sparkle. There were many other excellent humans in the ABC who contributed brain power, strategic vision, heart, audio craft or editorial nous to that pilot season, including Angela Stengel, Linda Bracken, Jo Upham, Judith Whelan, Amanda Armstrong, Selena Shannon, Judy Rapley, Brigit Berger, Andrew Davies, Justine Kelly, Deb Leavitt, Angela Owens, Joel Werner, Jonathan Webb and Ian Walker. A special thank you to Scott Spark for introducing us (Yumi and Claudine) and seeing the potential that might come from *Ladies*. We'll be forever grateful to the team who took the baton for season two of the podcast and made it even more special. Cassandra Steeth, Madeleine Genner, Monique Bowley and Justine Kelly – what a cracking job you all did.

Emily Hart, our commissioning editor from Hardie Grant Books, you are a saint. Thanks for helping us create a vision for exactly what this book might be and being a calm guiding force as we realised that vision. We really don't know how you managed to do that while living through six lockdowns and umpteen rewrites. Grace Lee's illustrations and Reg Abos's design brought the pages to life. We'd also like to acknowledge the rest of the book team and those at Hardie Grant who have been supportive, thoughtful and encouraging at every turn.

Cassandra Steeth and Tahnee Jash, thanks for the long phone calls on how we make sure this book is as inclusive as possible, and then helping to find the voices of those who were missing. Lisa Hunter from ABC Commercial, we genuinely appreciate that you wrangled permissions and paperwork so that we didn't have to. Justine Kelly, we're not sure how you found the time to read through and give thoughtful feedback on several different rounds of edits, but you're living testament to what they say about giving jobs to busy women.

Thank you to all of the experts who featured in the podcast and now this book, and a special acknowledgement to Tanya Koens, Dr Gemma Sharp, Dr Melissa Kang, Dr Deb Bateson, Cass Dunn and Dr Rosie Worsley, who kindly took the time to review pages for us.

CLAUDINE

I'm incredibly grateful to Yumi for responding to my text back in 2017. I have never felt so outside my comfort zone as I have since we started working together, and I wouldn't change it for a second. I feel so bloody lucky to have you in my life.

I have always been drawn to real conversations, the ones that involve laughter, sometimes tears, and that end because you run out of time, not things to say. Among my nearest and dearest are many wonderful women who are up for this kind of conversation and have taught me that some of the greatest gifts you can give someone are your time, attention and a safe space to talk. So, a special thank you to my mum Jan, step-mum Helen, my mother-in-law Pam, my aunties – Paula, Sandra, Jule, Trish – and many darling friends, including Emma, Lesley, Laura, Kirrin, Megan, Christy, Claire, Fiona, Thea, Pia, Libby, Nic, Michelle, Ariel, Sonya, Tegan (both of you), Genelle, Angela, Mon, Kylie, Ginger, Edwina, Jazz, Caroline, Alex, Beth, Candice, Julieanne and Felicity.

While I'm drawn to the conversations that happen in safe places for women and gender-diverse people, most of close relatives are male and I love them dearly. Blake, thank you for supporting and encouraging me always, especially during the tough times and moments of self-doubt. My darling sons Parker and Ruben, thanks for the endless cups of tea, listening to me talk about things you'd rather not hear from your mother and believing in me when I lose confidence in myself. Finally, to my youngest, precious curly-haired son Atticus Django, thank you for helping me to write these acknowledgements and genuinely believing that this is a very important book.

★

YUMI

I'd like to thank the coronavirus for being such a massive asshole that it's created a real benchmark against which all future assholes will be measured. Fuck you. I owe a huge debt of thanks to Gerard Cain and family, particularly Chris Cain and Madeline Ybarzabal, for letting me use their island home to work in while things around us crumbled to dust. My friends, Lisa BBQ, Carla, Jade, Marihuzka, Cass, Penny A, Dr Melissa Kang, Katie Dimond, Mel Davies, and the beloved bozos I run with, Ben P, Lisa F, Celine, Sarah H, Jaime and Andy – if I am a prolapse waiting to happen, you people are the pelvic floor that supports me, the scaffolding that stops me slipping through and spattering onto the floor in a mess of gunk and despair. Thanks to Marisa Pintado for knowing there was life in *Ladies, We Need To Talk* beyond a podcast. Finally, Claudine Ryan, thanks for being a sister, confidante, enthusiastic learner, listener and friend. You know how they say 'You've gotta do the work'? You're always doing the work. Let's hold hands and watch as the world burns.

Published in 2021 by Hardie Grant Books,
an imprint of Hardie Grant Publishing

Hardie Grant Books (Melbourne)
Wurundjeri Country
Building 1, 658 Church Street
Richmond, Victoria 3121

Hardie Grant Books (London)
5th & 6th Floors
52–54 Southwark Street
London SE1 1UN

hardiegrantbooks.com

 A catalogue record for this
book is available from the
National Library of Australia

Ladies, We Need To Talk
ISBN 978 1 74379 751 8

10 9 8 7 6 5 4 3 2 1

Design by Regine Abos
Printed in Australia by Griffin Press, part of Ovato, an Accredited ISO AS/
NZS 14001 Environmental Management System printer.

 The paper this book is printed on is certified against the
Forest Stewardship Council® Standards. Griffin Press holds
FSC® chain of custody certification SGSHK-COC-005088. FSC®
promotes environmentally responsible, socially beneficial and
economically viable management of the world's forests.

Hardie Grant acknowledges the Traditional Owners of the country
on which we work, the Wurundjeri people of the Kulin nation and the
Gadigal people of the Eora nation, and recognises their continuing
connection to the land, waters and culture. We pay our respects to their
Elders past, present and emerging.